PHYSICAL DIAGNOSIS
IN MEDICINE

PHYSICAL DIAGNOSIS IN MEDICINE

A E DAVIS
M.D.(Syd.), M.A., B.Sc.(Oxon.), M.R.C.P., M.R.A.C.P.
Associate Professor in Medicine, University of
New South Wales, Sydney, Australia

T D BOLIN
M.D.(N.S.W.), M.R.C.P., M.R.C.P.(Ed.), F.R.A.C.P., D.C.H.
Senior Lecturer in Medicine, University of
New South Wales, Sydney, Australia

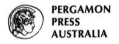

**PERGAMON
PRESS
AUSTRALIA**

Pergamon Press (Australia) Pty Ltd
19a Boundary Street, Rushcutters Bay, NSW 2011

Pergamon Press Ltd
Headington Hill Hall, Oxford OX3 OBW

Pergamon Press Inc.
Fairview Park, Elmsford, NY 10523

Pergamon of Canada Ltd
207 Queen's Quay West, Toronto 1

Vieweg & Sohn
GmbH, Burgplatz 1, Braunschweig, West Germany

First Published 1973

Cover design by Vane Lindesay

Typeset in Australia by Acet Pty Ltd, Rushcutters Bay, NSW 2011

Printed in Hong Kong by Wing King Tong Co Ltd

National Library of Australia Card Number and ISBN 0 08 017376 4

CONTENTS

Acknowledgements

Preface

ACKNOWLEDGEMENTS

In writing this book we acknowledge the debt owed to the many teachers who stimulated our interest in Clinical Medicine and to the students who have maintained it.

We are indebted to Professor R. B. Blacket, Foundation Professor of Medicine, The University of New South Wales, Sydney, for his continued advice and encouragement and in particular for his careful criticism of the manuscript.

We are also grateful to Dr P. Brennan & Dr D. Gillies, and other members of the School of Medicine, Prince Henry Hospital, Sydney, for their helpful criticisms.

We are grateful to Mrs B. Whearty and Mrs P. Cremonesi for typing the manuscript and to Mr K. Deason, Mr G. Thompson, Penny Zylstra and Robin Bolin for the illustrations.

PREFACE

The objectives of this book are to enable the student to carry out a physical examination, to give the common causes of abnormal physical signs, and to outline the physical signs encountered in common medical conditions.

We have deliberately refrained from giving exhaustive lists of causes for conditions described. For example, when discussing jaundice six common causes are given which together account for over 95 per cent of all cases. The rare causes omitted can in most instances only be diagnosed by using ancillary aids and consequently are beyond the scope of this book.

At times rare causes are included in a differential diagnosis as in these cases the physical signs described may be the clue to the definitive diagnosis. For example, constrictive pericarditis even though rare, is included in the differential diagnosis of atrial fibrillation, as in this instance unexplained atrial fibrillation may alert the physician to the possible diagnosis.

A. E. DAVIS

T. D. BOLIN

PRELIMINARY APPRAISAL OF THE PATIENT

The first meeting of the physician with the patient is important in that a mutual appraisal of each other is made. The physician's initial appraisal takes note of the patient's demeanour and dress, as this may relate subsequently to the content of the history. At the same time some insight is gained into the patient's educational and social background. His general behaviour and mood may be affected by the underlying disorder or may be altered by his reaction to it. For example, the patient with thyrotoxicosis may be agitated and apprehensive; however, a similar mental state can be produced by the patient's anxiety regarding his underlying illness. It should also be remembered that such an anxiety state need not necessarily be associated with underlying organic disease. While a serious organic disorder may not be reflected in the appearance of the patient, evidence of recent weight loss and an appearance of ill-health should alert the physician to the possibility of a serious underlying disease.

During this general appraisal of the patient a number of important physical signs may be evident.

PALLOR AND PLETHORA

Anaemia usually can be detected clinically when the haemoglobin level falls below 11.0 gm per 100 ml blood and at this stage there will be pallor of the conjunctivae, face and palms of the hands. With more severe degrees of anaemia the palmar creases lose their normal pink colouration signifying a haemoglobin value of less than 8.0 gm per 100 ml of blood (page 92). If conjunctival pallor is absent, facial pallor does not signify anaemia. Similarly facial plethora does not necessarily signify polycythaemia. The observation of pallor or plethora warrants a haemoglobin estimation.

CYANOSIS

This is a bluish discolouration of the skin and mucous membranes associated with an increase in the reduced haemoglobin concentration in the underlying blood vessels. Cyanosis may be:

1. **Central**

   The cyanosis is observed in warm areas such as the tongue and mucous membranes of the inner surfaces of the lips. That the tongue is in fact warm requires confirmation by palpation.
   Causes
   i. Right to left cardiac shunts associated with cyanotic congenital heart disease or other pulmonary arterio-venous shunts.
   ii. Pulmonary disease − obstructive airways disease including obstruction to the trachea or major bronchi; defects of pulmonary diffusion and perfusion, e.g., pulmonary oedema, pneumonia and interstitial fibrosis.
   iii. Depression of the respiratory centre by drugs or raised intra-cranial pressure.
   iv. Methaemoglobinaemia and sulphaemoglobinaemia.

2. **Peripheral**

   The cyanosis occurs in the extremities, including the outer surface of the lips, nose and ears, these areas being cold. It is not always easy to differentiate central from peripheral cyanosis.
   Causes
   i. Peripheral vascular disease (small vessels)
   ii. Cardiac failure
   iii. Hypothermia.

PIGMENTATION

Pigmentation occurs both in the skin and mucous membranes and while it may be more evident in areas normally exposed to the sun it should be apparent in other areas such as the inner aspect of the forearms. Pigmentation is commonly racial in origin, associated with exposure to the sun, and occurs in pregnancy. However, certain disease states are associated with pigmentation.

1. Addison's disease
2. Haemochromatosis
3. Cirrhosis of the liver
4. Uraemia
5. Thyrotoxicosis
6. Malignant lymphomas and carcinomas
7. Malabsorption syndromes
8. Cachexia
9. Acanthosis nigricans
10. Drugs e.g. bromides and heavy metals.

JAUNDICE

This is best observed in natural light and is first apparent in the sclerae, when the bilirubin level will be more than 1.5 mg per 100 ml of blood. It may in fact not be apparent in artificial light till the level of bilirubin rises much higher. In long-standing cholestatic jaundice there is a greenish tinge to the jaundice which may be associated with xanthomas, bruising and pruritis. Haemolytic jaundice is usually slight and may be associated with anaemia. Hepatocellular jaundice may be associated with stigmata of chronic liver disease.

Causes

i. Hepatitis
     Infectious, including mononucleosis
     Alcoholic
ii. Gallstones
iii. Carcinoma of the pancreas

iv. Cirrhosis of the liver
v. Drugs
vi. Haemolysis.

SPOT DIAGNOSIS

It may be possible during the initial appraisal of the patient to make a spot diagnosis as there are a number of conditions which have characteristic features. These include thyrotoxicosis, myxoedema, acromegaly, Cushing's disease and syndrome, hypopituitarism, uraemia, nephrotic syndrome, Parkinson's disease and the myopathies.

Furthermore, there are typical facial appearances such as the malar flush associated with mitral valve disease, the butterfly rash of disseminated lupus erythematosis, and the alcoholic facies comprising puffiness, parotid enlargement and multiple telangiectasia.

EXAMINATION OF THE HANDS

Before proceeding to a systematic physical examination it is pertinent to examine the hands, as they may show evidence of systemic disorders. The changes detected include:

Generalised enlargement

In acromegaly a generalised enlargement including both the soft tissues and bones occurs. Long thin fingers (arachnodactyly) occur as a component of Marfan's syndrome.

Clubbing of the fingers

There is obliteration of the angle at the junction of the base of the nail and the skin of the terminal phalanx; this may be associated with curvature of the tip of the nail (beaking), and enlargement of the end of the finger (drumstick). Similar appearances may be present in the toes.

Causes
i. *Conditions above the diaphragm*

a. Pulmonary

    Carcinoma of the lung

    Long-standing lung infections e.g. pulmonary abscess and tuberculosis

b. Cardiovascular

    Cyanotic congenital heart disorders

    Subacute bacterial endocarditis

ii. *Conditions below the diaphragm*

    Cirrhosis of the liver

    Chronic diarrhoeas including steatorrhoea and ulcerative colitis

iii. *Thyrotoxicosis*

iv. *Congenital*

v. *Idiopathic.*

Pulmonary hypertrophic osteoarthropathy, occurring in carcinoma of the lung, consists of clubbing of the fingers, associated with rheumatoid-like changes in the hands and wrists.

Palmar erythema

A reddish mottling occurring in the skin over the thenar and hypothenar eminences of the hands and associated with:

1. Chronic liver disease
2. Rheumatoid arthritis
3. Collagen disorders
4. Thyrotoxicosis
5. Pregnancy
6. Normality.

Wasting of the small muscles of the hands

There are 20 intrinsic muscles in the hand, 15 of them are innervated by the ulnar nerve and 5 by the median (thenar eminence). All the intrinsic muscles are innervated by the T 1 nerve root.

In the presence of wasting of the small muscles of the hand the metacarpal bones are prominent and on firmly adducting the thumb there is absence of the normal prominence of the first interosseous muscle. This wasting also affects the thenar and hypothenar eminences and may be best appreciated by palpation.

Causes

i. Anterior horn cell lesions
      Motor neurone disease
      Syringomyelia
      Spinal cord tumours
ii. Peripheral neuropathy
iii. Cervical rib
iv. Lesions of the median and ulnar nerves
v. Dystrophia myotonica
vi. Arthritis.

Dupuytren's contracture

A localised thickening of the palmar fascia which may produce contractures of the flexor tendons, beginning initially on the ulnar side of the hands. It can occur in normal subjects, but when it occurs in association with liver disease it signifies an alcoholic aetiology for that liver disease.

Heberden's nodes

Localised bony swellings occurring on the sides of the dorsum of the distal interphalangeal joints, particularly in women in whom there may be a family history.

Nails

A common abnormality is brittleness occurring particularly in women, and often associated with the use of detergents. However, brittleness frequently occurs in thyrotoxicosis and iron deficiency where it may be associated with spoon shaped nails (koilonychia). Longitudinal haemorrhages occurring under the tips of the nails (sub-ungual haemorrhages) are commonly associated with trauma, but classically occur in subacute bacterial endocarditis. Pitting of the nails occurs with psoriasis, which may be associated with a rheumatoid-like arthritis which is distinguished by the fact that the terminal interphalangeal joints are involved (psoriatic arthropathy). These joints are unaffected in classical rheumatoid arthritis.

Arthritis (page 117)

2

THE NERVOUS SYSTEM

At the first interview with the patient an assessment is made of his appearance, behaviour and mental state, realising that factors such as poor understanding of English, deafness, dysphasia and sedation may affect this assessment. The following is an outline of a schematic approach which allows an overall assessment to be made.

APPEARANCE AND GENERAL BEHAVIOUR

The following are noted.
1. Does the patient look ill?
2. Is he in touch with his surroundings and are his relationships with the staff and other patients normal?
3. Does he make any abnormal gestures, grimaces or other motor movements?
4. Do these movements and attitudes have any evident purpose?

Talk

The patient's approach to conversation is assessed and some insight into his educational background obtained. Does he say much or little, talk spontaneously or require prompting; is his conversation coherent; are there sudden silences or changes of topic and are his comments relevant? If his talk is inappropriate this could be due to:

1. Psychological abnormality
2. Organic impairment of cerebral function
3. General disturbances such as thyrotoxicosis or myxoedema.
   Samples of the patient's abnormal talk should be recorded.

Mood

The general appearance of the patient may reflect his underlying mood. However, the response to a question such as, "How do you feel in yourself?" allows a better assessment. It is important to allow the patient time to express himself. Many varieties of mood may be present, not merely happiness or sadness, but states such as irritability, suspicion, fear, unreality, worry, restlessness, bewilderment and many more. The relevance of the patient's apparent emotional state to his symptomatology is important.

Orientation

If appropriate, a record of the patient's answers to questions about his name, identity, the place where he is, the time of day and date, including the month and the year, should be made.

Memory

This is tested by comparing the patient's account of his life to that given by others. There should be special enquiry regarding events such as those of his admission to hospital and subsequent happenings in the ward. Where there is selective impairment of memory for special incidents, and recent or remote happenings, this should be recorded in detail and the patient's attitude towards his forgetfulness also recorded. An assessment of recent memory can be made by telling the patient a short story which contains five facts; the patient is then asked to recall these five facts or repeat the story five minutes later.

Insight and judgment

What is the patient's attitude to his present state? Does he regard it as an illness which needs treatment? Is he aware of mistakes made spontaneously or in response to tests? How does he regard them and other details of his condition? What is his attitude towards social, financial and ethical problems? Is his judgment good? What does he propose to do when he has left hospital?

All the above facts will not be obtained during the patient's first interview, but become apparent during his stay in hospital or in further interviews.

Handedness

It should be noted whether the patient is right or left handed as this will usually indicate the dominant hemisphere and thus have a direct relationship to disorders of speech.

Speech

It is important that the patient understands the purpose of the tests and these should be explained to him in appropriate terms.

1. *Dysphasia*

This is a disturbance of language and the following varieties occur.

   i. *Inability to understand spoken words — sensory aphasia* (left temporo-parietal region). This is assessed by giving the patient a series of commands which gradually increase in difficulty such as "close your eyes", "touch your right ear", "touch your right ear with the index finger of the right hand".

   ii. *Inability to understand written words — dyslexia* (left parieto-occipital region). A series of written commands is given to the patient in order of increasing complexity, e.g. "open your mouth", "put your hand on top of your head", "touch your right ear with your left thumb".

   iii. *Inability to select words and name objects — motor or nominal aphasia* (left inferior frontal and left temporo-parietal regions). The patient is asked to name a series of common objects. Often the patient may name objects used frequently, e.g. cup, spoon; but may have difficulty with objects that are used infrequently, e.g. buckle, winder of a watch, watch strap. When the aphasia is severe the patient may be unable to utter a word.

iv. *Inability to write — agraphia* (left temporo-parietal region). The patient is asked to write an account of the events occurring during the morning.

2. **Dysarthria**

This is a disorder of articulation, in contrast to dysphasia which is a disorder of language. The following varieties occur.

i. *Cerebellar.* A scanning or slurred speech in which the words are broken up into syllables.

ii. *Extra-pyramidal.* The speech is slow and monotonous and the voice is soft.

iii. *Bulbar palsy.* This produces a nasal type of speech.

iv. *Drugs.* A slurred speech is produced by sedatives such as alcohol and barbiturates.

Dyspraxia

Dyspraxia is an inability to perform tasks in the absence of weakness, sensory loss or impaired cerebellar function, and commonly occurs in left parietal or frontal lobe lesions. The patient is given a packet of cigarettes and a box of matches and is asked to light a cigarette; or is asked to use a pair of scissors, a comb or a pencil.

The following is a scheme outlining the physical examination of the nervous system.

THE SKULL

This is inspected and palpated for any underlying bony or soft tissue abnormality. Auscultation is carried out over the mastoids, temples and orbits. During auscultation over the orbits the stethoscope is placed over one eye, the other eye is opened and the patient is asked to stop breathing. Auscultation is then carried out over the carotid arteries with the patient holding his breath.

THE SPINE

Any deformity, tenderness or limitation of movement of the cervical, thoracic or lumbar spine is noted.

CRANIAL NERVES

FIRST CRANIAL NERVE (OLFACTORY)

Anatomy

The first cranial nerve is sensory and arises from receptors in the mucous membrane of the nose. The fibres pass through the cribriform plate of the ethmoid to the olfactory bulb, forming the olfactory tract and terminating in the temporal lobes.

Examination

A simple test for smell is to ask the patient if his sense of smell is normal. Loss of smell is rarely of neurological importance as it is usually due to a nasal lesion. To detect unilateral anosmia the patient occludes one nostril with his index finger and his ability to distinguish various odours with the other nostril is assessed.

Causes of unilateral anosmia

i.   Fracture of the anterior fossa
ii. Meningioma of the olfactory groove or sphenoidal ridge
iii. Basal meningitis.

SECOND CRANIAL NERVE (OPTIC NERVE)

Anatomy

The fibres of the optic nerve originate in the ganglion cells of the retina and converge towards the optic disc, penetrating the lamina cribrosa to form the optic nerve which passes through the optic foramen in association with the ophthalmic artery. At the base of the brain fibres of the two nerves join to form the optic chiasma. In the optic nerve the fibres from the upper retina lie superiorly and those from the lower part lie inferiorly. In the optic chiasma the fibres from the nasal half of the retina (from the temporal visual fields) decussate, whereas those from the temporal part of the retina (from the nasal visual field) do not. The fibres concerned with vision then travel in the optic tract to the lateral geniculate body and thence by the optic radiation through the posterior limb of the internal capsule to the occipital pole. Fibres concerned with the light reflex terminate in the superior colliculus from where connections are made with both third nerve nuclei. The fibres in the right optic tract carry visual impulses from the temporal half of the right retina and the nasal half of the left retina and constitute the left homonymous visual field. A similar arrangement exists in the optic radiation. The macula has bilateral cortical representation.

Examination
Visual acuity
This is assessed by asking the patient to read a passage from a newspaper with one eye, the other being closed. If a visual defect is found more formal testing can be performed using a Snellen's chart. This chart should be used to record visual acuity in patients with suspected intra-cranial disease in order to detect subsequent changes.
Visual fields
These are tested by confrontation, with the examiner sitting about three feet from the patient. The examiner's arms are extended with the fingers midway between the examiner and the patient, who is asked to look at the examiner's nose. Small movements of the fingers are made at the periphery of the examiner's field of vision and the patient's peripheral vision is assessed by asking him to point to the finger which moved. If an abnormality is detected then the defect is delineated using either the same method or a small white pin head. More detailed assessment necessitates a Bjerrum's screen.
The light reflex
The pupils are inspected to determine if they are regular in contour and equal in diameter. The light reflex is elicited by shining a torch onto the pupil, taking care to approach from the side of the eye. A normal direct reflex results in constriction of the pupil on that side. A consensual or indirect light reflex occurs when the pupil of the other eye also constricts. The reaction of the pupils to accommodation is observed by asking the patient to focus on an approaching object such as the examiner's index finger. The pupils will constrict as the eyes converge.

Ophthalmoscopy

It is advisable to have a good personal ophthalmoscope. The patient should be examined sitting or standing, fixing his gaze on a distant object. To observe the right fundus the examiner holds the ophthalmoscope up to his right eye, ensuring that his head is upright and not occluding the vision of the patient's left eye. If this is not done the patient will be unable to fix his gaze and will focus on the examiner's head thus constricting the pupil and making the examination difficult. Examine the cornea, pupil and the iris starting with a 20+ lens and changing the lenses until the retina is in focus. The disc can be found by identifying a vessel and tracing it centrally. Ophthalmoscopy is ideally performed after the pupils have been dilated with homatropine.

Examination of the disc

Colour. This is normally whitish, the temporal side being a shade paler than the nasal. An abnormally white disc indicates optic atrophy. Unilateral atrophy may be best appreciated by rapidly comparing both discs. An abnormally pink disc suggests papilloedema or papillitis.

Contour. The temporal margins are usually sharply defined, whereas the nasal margins may be slightly blurred. Increased blurring of the nasal margin occurs early in papilloedema.

The optic cup and lamina cribrosa. In the normal disc the physiological cup and lamina cribrosa can be identified. The cup is obliterated in papilloedema and secondary optic atrophy, whereas it is accentuated in primary optic atrophy and glaucoma.

Circulation. This is examined by identifying the superior and inferior temporal and nasal arteries and veins and following each from the disc to the periphery. Normally the veins are slightly larger than the arteries (a ratio of 3:2). The centre of the arteries appears lighter than the periphery (the light reflex), and in arterial disease this may be increased and may be associated with arterial tortuosity. Distension of the veins occurs in papilloedema and may be more readily detected than early swelling of the disc. If the retinal veins are not distended then papilloedema is not present.

Retina and choroid. Such abnormalities as haemorrhages, exudates, oedema and the changes of choroiditis are noted. The changes of choroiditis appear behind a normal retinal circulation, thus being distinguished from retinitis.

Lesions detected during examination of the second cranial nerve

1. *Interruption of the visual pathways*
   i. Lesions of the optic nerve result in unilateral blindness.
   ii. Lesions to the central part of the chiasma produce bitemporal hemianopia, e.g. pituitary tumours.
   iii. Complete lesions of the optic tract produce an homonymous hemianopia with preservation of the direct light reflex.
   iv. Lesions of the optic radiation are more usually incomplete than complete owing to its wide radiation, and result in partial homonymous hemianopia.

2. *Papilloedema*
   Physical signs are blurring of the disc margins and obliteration of the physiological cup and lamina cribrosa, retinal oedema and dilated retinal veins.
   Causes
   a. Raised intracranial pressure
   b. Hypertension (severe)
   c. Thrombosis of the central retinal vein
   d. Retrobulbar neuritis involving the nerve head
   e. Superior vena-caval obstruction.

3. *Secondary optic atrophy*
   This follows long-standing papilloedema and is manifest by pallor of the optic disc with an ill-defined physiological cup and lamina cribrosa.

4. *Primary optic atrophy*
   The disc is pale with a normal physiological cup and lamina cribrosa. It is associated with some impairment of visual acuity.

Causes

a. The causes of retrobulbar neuritis
b. Pressure by tumours in the region of the optic nerve and chiasma
c. In association with hereditary and familial ataxias
d. Associated with retinitis pigmentosa.

5. *Retrobulbar neuritis*

This is characterised by blurring of vision and a visual field defect, usually a central scotoma; a dilated pupil which has a sluggish direct light reflex and a normal consensual light reflex; papilloedema may be associated (papillitis).

Causes

a. Disseminated sclerosis
b. Neurosyphilis
c. Chemical poisons — methyl alcohol, tobacco, etc.
d. Neuromyelitis optica
e. Vitamin B.12 deficiency.

6. *Retinopathy*

The two common medical conditions affecting the retina are:

i. *Hypertension.* The arteries are narrow, tortuous, have an increased light reflex and compress the veins at points of crossing (A-V nipping). Haemorrhages may occur and are usually flame shaped and may be associated with fluffy exudates which in later stages become hard and discrete, particularly around the macula (macular star). Papilloedema may also occur. A classification involving grading need not be used; any abnormalities seen should be accurately described and drawn in a sketch so that subsequent changes can be easily recognised.

Retinal haemorrhages imply necrotising arteritis in the kidneys. Accelerated hypertension is indicated by the presence of fresh haemorrhages or exudates and papilloedema.

ii. *Diabetes.* Characteristic retinal changes are "dot" and "blot" haemorrhages and exudates occurring particularly towards the periphery and adjacent to vessels. Micro-aneurysms have a similar distribution. As diabetes and hypertension frequently coexist the retinal changes often overlap.

7. *Choroiditis*

This appears as white patches occurring behind the retinal vessels and often associated with discrete black pigmentation.

Causes

a. Toxoplasmosis
b. Sarcoidosis
c. Trauma
d. Syphilis
e. Tuberculosis
f. Idiopathic.

A textbook of ophthalmology should be consulted for the following important conditions.

Retinal vein thrombosis, central and branch
Embolism of the central retinal artery
Leukaemic retinopathy
Medullated nerve fibres
Retinitis pigmentosa
Subhyaloid haemorrhage.

THE THIRD, FOURTH AND SIXTH CRANIAL NERVES

THE THIRD CRANIAL NERVE (OCULOMOTOR)

Anatomy

The nucleus, in fact a collection of nuclei, is situated in the upper part of the mid-brain. The fibres pass through the mid-brain into the posterior fossa where they are in close relationship to the posterior cerebral and superior cerebellar vessels. The nerve then crosses the middle fossa in the wall of the cavernous sinus in association with the fourth, the ophthalmic division of the fifth and the sixth cranial nerves, these nerves leaving the skull together through the superior orbital fissure. The third nerve supplies all the ocular muscles except the superior oblique and external rectus. In addition it supplies the levator palprebrae superioris and the sphincter pupillae.

THE FOURTH CRANIAL NERVE (TROCHLEAR)

Anatomy

The fourth nerve originates in the mid-brain and accompanies the third nerve in the cavernous sinus, supplying the superior oblique muscle.

THE SIXTH CRANIAL NERVE (ABDUCENS)

Anatomy

The sixth nerve originates in the pons leaving between the anterior inferior cerebellar artery and the internal auditory artery. It passes laterally in the cerebello-pontine angle and then anteriorly over the petrous temporal bone where it is in close association with the fifth nerve. The nerve proceeds forwards and medially to the cavernous sinus leaving the skull through the superior orbital fissure and supplying the external rectus muscle.

Examination of the third, fourth and sixth cranial nerves

The functions of the three nerves are tested together as follows.

1. *Ptosis*

   A drooping of the upper eyelid which may be unilateral or bilateral, partial or complete. Normally the upper lid comes half way between the upper border of the iris and the pupil while the lower lid comes to the lower border of the iris.

   Causes

   a. Third nerve palsy. Associated signs are a fixed dilated pupil and ophthalmoplegia.
   b. Seventh nerve lesion — associated with obvious facial weakness.
   c. Interruption of the sympathetic nervous supply (Horner's syndrome). Ptosis is never complete.
   d. Myopathy. e.g., myaesthenia gravis, dystrophia myotonica. The ptosis is bilateral and incomplete.
   e. Congenital. Usually bilateral, never complete and not associated with other neurological signs.
   f. Tabes dorsalis. Bilateral, never complete and may be associated with Argyll Robertson pupils.

2. *Ophthalmoplegia and diplopia*

To detect ophthalmoplegia the patient sits confronting the examiner who steadies the patient's hand with one hand while a finger of the other hand is held at least 20 inches from the head and moved through the full range of ocular movements.

Differentiation of the false from the true image is often possible using the following criteria:

i. The separation of the images is greatest when the affected muscle is in use

ii. The more peripheral image is always the false image

iii. The false image disappears when the affected eye is covered.

Unless the upper lids are retracted while testing downward gaze abnormalities will be missed. Any abnormalities of ocular movement are noted and the patient is asked to indicate whether diplopia occurs, as it may be present without detectable ophthalmoplegia.

The ophthalmoplegia of a complete third nerve lesion causes the eye to look laterally and downwards due to the unopposed action of the lateral rectus and the superior oblique, whereas a lesion of the sixth nerve causes the eye to deviate medially due to the weakness of the external rectus muscle. An isolated lesion of the fourth cranial nerve is rare.

3. *Nystagmus*

Involuntary, oscillating and rhythmical movements of the eyes which may be present at rest but are accentuated by conjugate deviation of the eyes. Nystagmus is looked for while examining ocular movements, the examiner ensuring that his finger does not go beyond the field of binocular vision as this may cause nystagmus in normal subjects. Phasic nystagmus has two components, usually quicker in one direction than in the other — the quick and slow phases. The direction of the nystagmus is taken from the direction of the quick phase. Thus, if the quick phase is to the right the patient is said to have nystagmus to the right. Nystagmus may be present when the eyes look straight ahead, but is usually accentuated by conjugate deviation of the eyes.

Causes

a. Lesions of the cerebellum and its connections within the brainstem. The nystagmus is phasic and often most marked on conjugate deviation to the side of the lesion. Nystagmus which occurs on upward or downward conjugate gaze indicates a brainstem lesion.

b. Lesions of the labyrinths. These also produce a phasic nystagmus, often with a rotary component, which may be precipitated by sudden movements of the head and is often difficult to distinguish from cerebellar nystagmus.

c. Visual. Occurs in association with severe congenital amblyopia. The movements of the eyes are pendular.

4. *Pupils*

The size, shape, symmetry and the response to light and accommodation are noted. Pupil size is dependent upon the interaction between the sympathetic component supplying the dilator pupillae and the para-sympathetic component which accompanies the third nerve and supplies the sphincter pupillae. The reaction to light and accommodation has been described (page 12).

Abnormalities

i. *Small pupils*

a. Pin-point regular pupils occur with pontine haemorrhage, drugs such as morphine and interruption of the sympathetic pathway (Horner's syndrome).

b. Argyll Robertson pupils (neurosyphilis). Bilateral, small, irregular, unequal pupils which do not react to light but react briskly to accommodation and associated with patchy depigmentation or the iris.

ii. *Large pupils*

a. Third nerve lesions

b. Drugs such as cocaine and homatropine.

iii. *Irregular pupils*

The commonest cause is iritis.

Lesions of the third and sixth cranial nerves

Causes of a third nerve paralysis

All cranial nerves may be affected in their intra-cerebral, extra-cerebral and extra-cranial pathways by similar conditions. The following scheme can be suitably applied to other cranial nerves.

i. *Nucleus and mid brain*
   a. Disseminated sclerosis
   b. Neoplasms
   c. Vascular lesions.

   The deficit is frequently bilateral, incomplete and rarely isolated due to the proximity of other structures. A third nerve paralysis associated with upper motor neurone signs on the opposite side localises the lesion to the mid brain.

ii. *Posterior fossa*
   a. Fracture of the base of the skull
   b. Aneurysm of the posterior communicating artery
   c. Neurosyphilis
   d. Basal meningitis.

   The signs are unilateral and may occur without other cranial nerves being involved.

iii. *Cavernous sinus*
   a. Thrombosis associated with infection
   b. Aneurysm of the internal carotid artery.

   The signs are unilateral and often associated with those of a lesion of the fourth, ophthalmic division of the fifth and sixth nerves. Cavernous sinus thrombosis may also produce exophthalmos, chemosis and papilloedema which is usually initially unilateral and often later bilateral.

iv. *Orbital*
   a. Fractures of the skull
   b. Retro-orbital swellings – tumours, aneurysms.

   The signs are unilateral and often associated with proptosis.

Causes of a sixth nerve paralysis

The above scheme can be used to localise the cause of a sixth nerve paralysis. A nuclear lesion may be associated with an ipsilateral seventh nerve paralysis of lower motor neurone type and contralateral hemiplegia. A cause peculiar to the sixth nerve is osteomyelitis of the apex of the petrous temporal bone complicating otitis media and causing an isolated sixth nerve paralysis.

An isolated lesion of the fourth cranial nerve is rare and does not produce obvious signs.

THE FIFTH CRANIAL NERVE (TRIGEMINAL)

Anatomy

A motor and sensory nucleus lie in the pons. Fibres subserving touch and posture relay from this nucleus to form the trigeminothalamic tract. Fibres concerned with pain and temperature turn downwards through the medulla into the upper cervical cord terminating in the nucleus of the spinal tract. This explains how a lesion of the upper cord can cause dissociated anaesthesia in the face. The motor and sensory roots leave the pons in the cerebellopontine angle, traversing over the petrous portion of the temporal bone in the middle cranial fossa. From the Gasserian ganglion the three divisions of the sensory nerve arise. The ophthalmic division runs in the lateral wall of the cavernous sinus in association with the third nerve and supplies the skin of the forehead, cornea and conjunctivae. The maxillary division emerges from the infraorbital foramen to supply the skin over the maxillary region anterior to the ear, the upper teeth and gums and the mucous membranes of the palate and nasopharynx. The mandibular division runs with the motor route and leaves the skull via the foramen Ovale supplying the skin of the lower jaw, lower teeth and gums and buccal mucous membranes.

The motor division supplies the pterygoid, masseter and temporalis muscles.

Examination

Sensation is tested in the three major areas supplied by the sensory divisions of the fifth nerve, the forehead, cheek and lower jaw. The method of testing sensation is described under examination of the peripheral nervous system.

Corneal and conjunctival reflexes

These are tested using a fine wisp of cotton wool. The patient stares ahead and the cotton wool is brought in from the lateral side of the eye. In the normal patient blinking of both eyes follows stimulation of the cornea and conjunctiva. An absent conjunctival reflex may occur in functional disorders; however, an absent corneal reflex always signifies organic disease and may be the earliest sign of involvement of the ophthalmic division of the fifth nerve. It is important to distinguish an absent corneal reflex due to a lesion of the fifth nerve from that due to a lesion of the seventh cranial nerve. A lesion of the fifth nerve results in an absence of blinking of both eyes when the affected side is tested. With a lesion of the seventh cranial nerve the blinking response is retained on the contralateral side, but is absent on the ipsilateral side due to weakness of the orbicularis oculi.

The temporal and masseter muscles are examined by inspection and palpation while the jaw is clenched. The pterygoids are examined by asking the patient to open his mouth. In the presence of weakness deviation of the jaw occurs towards the paralysed side due to the unopposed action of the opposite muscle. The jaw jerk is elicited by placing a finger on the chin of the half open jaw and striking firmly. An exaggerated jaw jerk indicates a bilateral upper motor neurone lesion above the pons.

Lesions of the fifth nerve produce wasting and weakness of the appropriate muscles, associated with sensory loss.

Lesions of the fifth nerve

In addition to disorders common to other cranial nerves there are further specific lesions.

1. Herpes Zoster

2. Trigeminal neuralgia
3. Otitis media
4. Acoustic neuroma.

THE SEVENTH CRANIAL NERVE (FACIAL)

Anatomy

This is a motor nerve with its nucleus in the pons in close proximity to the sixth cranial nerve. It leaves the pons in the cerebello-pontine angle entering the facial canal where it enlarges to form the geniculate ganglion. In the canal a branch is given off to the stapedius muscle; a lesion proximal to this branch will produce hyperacusis. The seventh nerve is then joined by the chorda tympani which subserves taste to the anterior half of the tongue. It leaves the facial canal through the stylomastoid foramen, passing through the parotid gland to supply the muscles of expression of the face, except the levator palpebrae superioris.

Examination

Minimal lesions of the seventh nerve are best appreciated during conversation. Lesions of the seventh cranial nerve are manifest by ipsilateral lack of wrinkling of the forehead, ptosis and drooping of the lower face which may not be obvious on inspection. When testing the facial muscles the patient is asked to wrinkle his forehead or frown; shut the eyes tightly and resist the examiner's attempt to open the closed eyes; puff out his cheeks, whistle and show his gums. Inability of the patient to bury his eyelashes on being asked to close the eyes tightly is an early sign of facial weakness.

Hyperacusis is best assessed by questioning the patient.

Facial paralysis can either be upper motor or lower motor neurone in type. Owing to the bilateral representation of the frontalis muscle in the cortex an upper motor neurone lesion produces weakness of the lower face with sparing of the forehead, while a lower motor neurone lesion produces weakness of both the upper and lower face.

Lesions of the seventh cranial nerve

In addition to the disorders common to other cranial nerves the following points should be noted.

1. Pontine lesions affecting the seventh nerve nucleus also involve the sixth nerve nucleus.
2. Cerebello-pontine angle lesions such as acoustic neuroma may affect the seventh, sixth and fifth cranial nerves.
3. Lesions at, or distal to, the stylomastoid foramen produce a lower motor neurone lesion with normal taste and hearing, whereas lesions in the facial canal may produce, in addition, hyperacusis and loss of taste in the anterior two thirds of the tongue.
4. Bilateral facial weakness is rare and if present is usually due to peripheral neuritis or muscular dystrophy.

Frequent causes of a seventh nerve lesion (lower motor neurone)

   i. Bell's palsy
   ii. Herpes Zoster. The typical vesicles being sought in the external auditory meatus
   iii. Surgery in the vicinity of the parotid gland.

THE EIGHTH CRANIAL NERVE (ACOUSTIC)

Anatomy

The eighth cranial nerve has two components subserving hearing and balance. Auditory fibres *(cochlear nerve)* arise from the organ of Corti in the inner ear and after a short course are joined by the fibres subserving balance *(vestibular nerve)* arising from the semicircular canals, forming the common eighth nerve which travels in the facial canal entering the cerebello-pontine angle through the internal auditory meatus. The auditory fibres enter the pons, partially decussate and have bilateral representation in the temporal cortices. Unilateral deafness from a central lesion is therefore not encountered. Vestibular fibres enter the pons and are widely distributed to the brain stem and cerebellum.

Examination

Lesions of this nerve produce disturbances of hearing and balance and are tested as follows.

1. *Hearing*

   The ears are initially inspected with the auriscope, the external meatus and the drum being visualised and the presence of wax noted. Hearing is tested with the opposite ear occluded by the examiner's finger. The patient is asked to repeat numbers whispered by the examiner who stands so that his lip movements cannot be seen. Alternatively the distance at which a ticking watch can be heard is recorded. If deafness is present then its type should be ascertained – conduction or nerve – by utilising the following tests.

   i. *Weber's test*

      A vibrating tuning fork is placed on the forehead in the mid-line. The sound is normally heard equally well in both ears. In conduction deafness the sound is localised to the affected ear while in nerve deafness it will be localised to the unaffected side.

   ii. *Rinne's test*

      A vibrating tuning fork is placed on the mastoid process, the patient indicating when it can no longer be heard. The fork is then placed at the external auditory meatus, the patient indicating whether the sound is now audible. Normally air conduction is better than bone conduction and the sound will again be heard. In nerve deafness, air conduction remains better than bone conduction whilst in conduction deafness bone conduction is better than air conduction. Unfortunately these two tests may give equivocal results.

2. *Balance*

   An ataxia may occur which is similar to that seen in cerebellar lesions (page 38). Lesions of the vestibular fibres may also be associated with vertigo and nystagmus. If nystagmus is not seen on routine testing then it may be provoked by sudden postural changes of the head. Refined testing of the semicircular canals is a specialist procedure and involves stimulation with hot and cold water.

Lesions of the eighth nerve

In addition to the disorders common to other cranial nerves the following should be noted.

1. Lesions of the external and the middle ear produce conduction deafness.
2. Involvement of the cochlear fibres outside the brain stem, e.g., acoustic neuroma, produces nerve deafness. Adjacent structures such as the fifth, sixth and seventh cranial nerves and brain stem (producing cerebellar and pyramidal signs) may be involved.
3. Impairment of balance may be caused by peripheral or central lesions. Common peripheral lesions are labyrinthitis, Ménière's disease, vestibular neuronitis, acoustic neuroma and drugs such as streptomycin and kanamycin.

NINTH AND TENTH CRANIAL NERVES (GLOSSOPHARYNGEAL AND VAGUS)

Anatomy

The ninth and tenth cranial nerves arise from nuclei situated in the medulla and leave the skull via the jugular foramen, supplying sensation to the posterior third of the tongue, the palate and upper pharynx and taste to the posterior third of the tongue. The vagus has further connections with the cardiovascular, pulmonary and gastro-intestinal systems, though these functions are not easily tested. The motor fibres supply the muscles of the palate, larynx and pharynx. These muscles have bilateral cortical representation and are therefore not affected by unilateral cerebral lesions. Unilateral paralysis is consequently of lower motor neurone type.

Examination

The palate is inspected and normally moves in the mid-line when the patient is asked to say "Ah". In the presence of palatal paralysis the palate moves upwards towards the unaffected side.

By stimulating the posterior pharyngeal wall a *gag reflex* is normally produced, this being a vigorous contraction of the upper pharyngeal muscles. The gag reflex is absent in a lower motor neurone lesion. The *palatal reflex* is tested by stimulation of the soft palate and observing its upward movement. Bilateral absence of the palatal reflex is not necessarily of clinical significance in that it may occur in functional disorders, while unilateral absence signifies a lower motor neurone lesion. In the presence of palatal paralysis dysphagia for fluids occurs, with regurgitation through the nose. A nasal voice is also present. Involvement of the recurrent laryngeal nerve produces hoarseness of the voice. Subsequent examination of the vocal cords requires a laryngoscope.

Lesions of the ninth and tenth cranial nerves

Unilateral lesions are often associated with involvement of the eleventh and twelfth cranial nerves and common causes are:
1. Naso-pharyngeal carcinoma
2. Fracture of the base of the skull
3. Paget's disease
4. Neoplasms near the jugular foramen.

Bilateral lesions may be either lower or upper motor neurone in type. In the presence of lower motor neurone lesions (true bulbar palsy), the eleventh and twelfth nerves are frequently involved and common causes are:
1. Motor neurone disease
2. Acute polyneuritis
3. Carcinoma of the naso-pharynx
4. Poliomyelitis.

Bilateral upper motor neurone lesions (pseudo-bulbar palsy) are commonly due to vascular lesions in the internal capsule producing a spastic dysarthria and bilateral pyramidal signs in the limbs.

THE ELEVENTH CRANIAL NERVE (SPINAL-ACCESSORY)

Anatomy

The eleventh nerve arises from widespread nuclei in the medulla and upper cervical cord and leaves the skull through the jugular foramen. The accessory division gives fibres to the vagus and the spinal division supplies the sternomastoid and trapezius muscles..

Examination

Inspection of the trapezius is carried out with the examiner standing behind the patient and palpating the trapezius while the patient shrugs his shoulders. To test the sternomastoid the examiner stands in front of the patient who rotates his head against the resistance of the examiner's hand against the jaw. The appropriate sternomastoid muscle is both inspected and palpated.

Lesions

These are similar to those discussed for the ninth and tenth cranial nerves.

THE TWELFTH CRANIAL NERVE (HYPOGLOSSAL)

Anatomy

The twelfth nerve arises from nuclei in the medulla and leaves the skull via the anterior condylar foramen which is adjacent to the jugular foramen. The twelfth cranial nerve supplies the muscles of the tongue.

Examination

The unprotruded tongue is inspected for the presence of fibrillation and wasting which occur in lower motor lesions. The tongue is then protruded and any deviation from the mid-line observed. Unilateral lesions of the twelfth nerve cause the tongue to deviate to the affected side, but solitary involvement is rare, the ninth, tenth and eleventh cranial nerves usually being affected (bulbar palsy). A small spastic tongue which is difficult to protrude is the result of a bilateral upper motor neurone lesion, pseudo-bulbar palsy.

EXAMINATION OF THE LIMBS AND TRUNK

The following scheme of examination is carried out.
1. Inspection for the presence of abnormal posture, involuntary movements, wasting and fasciculation
2. Assessment of tone
3. Assessment of power
4. Elicitation of the reflexes
5. Examination of sensation
6. Assessment of co-ordination

Abnormalities of posture are described in the section on neurological diagnosis (page 38).

Involuntary movements

Associated with involuntary movements may be alterations in posture which are dependent upon underlying tone. There are various forms of involuntary movements.

1. *Tremor*
    i. *Fine or physiological.* The patient is examined with the arms outstretched and the fingers apart. The tremor may be made more obvious if a sheet of paper is placed over the dorsum of the hands. The tremor is fine, rapid and accentuated by voluntary contraction. Such a tremor may be familial. Exaggeration of this tremor is common in Parkinson's disease and in emotional states including fatigue, thyrotoxicosis, senility and in association with drugs, including alcohol, nicotine, dexedrine, cocaine and heavy metals e.g., mercury.
    ii. *Extrapyramidal (Parkinsonism).* This tremor occurs at rest and may disappear on voluntary movement and during sleep and is increased by emotion. The tremor is coarse and rhythmical being typically "pill rolling" in the hand.

iii. *Cerebellar (Intention tremor)*. A coarse tremor accentuated by voluntary movements involving precision and absent at rest.

iv. *Metabolic (flapping tremor)*. The patient is asked to extend the arms, the wrists being hyper-extended with the fingers separated. The tremor consists of slow coarse and jerky movements of flexion and extension at the wrists through a wide arc. A fine tremor is often superimposed. A flapping tremor occurs in pre-hepatic coma, respiratory failure, uraemia and cardiac failure.

v. *A coarse tremor*. Involves the head, lips and tongue. It can occur in senility and cerebral syphilis or can be familial.

2. *Choreiform movements*

These movements are repetitive, quasi-purposeful and variable. They occur at rest, are involuntary, abrupt and brief and may be generalised or localised to any part of the body. They indicate an extra-pyramidal lesion.

3. *Athetoid movements*

These movements commonly occur at rest in association with choreiform movements and are involuntary, slow and writhing. They again indicate an extra-pyramidal lesion and may, like choreiform movements, be accentuated by voluntary movement and emotion.

4. *Tics*

These are repetitive, involuntary movements involving a localised area such as the face, and rarely associated with organic disease.

5. *Myoclonic jerks*

These are shock-like contractions of a muscle group which may displace a limb and are commonly associated with epilepsy.

6. *Hysterical movements*

These occur at rest or during voluntary movement and are bizarre, irregular and tend to diminish on distraction.

Wasting

This indicates a lower motor neurone lesion or myopathy and if associated with *fasciculation,* which is a visible twitching of groups of muscle fibres, indicates a progressive lesion involving the anterior horn cells. However, fasciculation in the absence of wasting or weakness is not pathological. Trophic changes frequently accompany wasting due to peripheral nerve lesions, and consist of smooth, thin, shiny, hairless skin and brittle nails.

Tone

Tone is assessed by gauging the resistance of the limb to passive movements; for example, in the upper limb, abduction and rotation of the shoulder; flexion and extension at the elbow; flexion, extension and rotation of the wrist. An increased resistance to passive movements indicates hypertonicity while decreased resistance to passive movements indicates hypotonicity. Assessment of tone is often difficult, particularly in the anxious patient who cannot relax.

Power

Power is assessed by the ability to overcome resistance and can be graded as follows:
0. No contraction
1. Flicker or trace of contraction
2. Active movement with gravity eliminated
3. Active movement against gravity
4. Active movement against resistance — degrees of resistance can be graded, 4.25, 4.50, 4.75
5. Normal power.

Method of examination

Flexors of the fingers

The examiner's and patient's flexed fingers are interlocked. The examiner attempts to overcome flexion.

Finger abduction

The patient widely abducts his fingers and the examiner attempts to close them with pressure over the proximal phalanges. Weakness thus detected may be the earliest sign of an upper motor neurone lesion.

Finger adduction

The fingers are firmly adducted against a piece of paper which is then withdrawn. Weakness is present with lesions affecting the intrinsic muscles of the hand.

Wrist extension

The patient extends his arm and cocks the wrist back. The examiner's hand grasps the lower forearm and base of the hand and attempts to overcome extension.

Wrist flexion

This rarely requires testing as weakness of wrist flexion does not occur in the absence of weakness of finger flexion.

Elbow flexion

The examiner attempts to overcome flexion of the elbow by grasping the patient's wrist, steadying the patient's arm at the elbow with his other hand.

Elbow extension

The patient attempts to extend the flexed elbow against the examiner's resistance applied at the wrist.

Shoulder abduction

The patient abducts the extended arm at least to the horizontal and the examiner, by pressing on the mid upper arm, attempts to overcome this abduction.

Reflexes

Radial jerk (C.5,6)

The patient's arms are relaxed, semi-pronated, flexed and rest on the thighs or abdomen. The lower end of the radius is struck with the reflex hammer and flexion of the arm observed.

Biceps jerk (C.5,6)

The arms are positioned as above, the examiner's thumb being placed over the tendon of the biceps and struck firmly. Contraction of the biceps is observed, producing flexion of the forearm.

Triceps jerk (C.7)

The patient rests the flexed forearm on his abdomen, the elbow being supported by the examiner. The tendon of the triceps is struck producing contraction of the muscle and resultant extension of the forearm.

The reflexes are recorded as follows.

	Right	**Left**
Radial jerk (C.5,6)	++	++
Biceps jerk (C.5,6)	++	++
Triceps jerk (C.7)	++	++

0   indicates absent reflexes
+   diminished reflexes
++   normal
+++ exaggerated reflexes.

Sensation

The patient is first asked whether any disturbance of sensation is present as formal methods of testing are relatively crude and will not elicit minor disturbances. The patient must understand what testing involves and this is best explained by demonstrating the appropriate sensation over a normal area such as the face. Testing is then carried out with the patient's eyes closed. Corresponding areas on both sides of the body are tested alternately and any areas of disturbed sensation are more carefully defined, moving from the abnormal area towards the normal. The following modalities of sensation are assessed.

Light touch

The skin is lightly touched with a wisp of cotton wool.

Pain

The skin is pricked with a pin, avoiding pressure.

Temperature

Hot and cold test tubes of water or a cold tuning fork are placed on the skin. Temperature rarely needs assessing unless a specific lesion such as syringomyelia is suspected.

Joint position sense

In the fingers this is tested by anchoring the middle phalanx with one hand and by gently holding the sides of the distal phalanx moving it through a range of passive movements. If any abnormality is detected larger joints such as the wrist or elbow are tested.

Vibration sense

In the upper limbs it is tested by applying the vibrating tuning fork (C 128) over the ulnar styloid process. If any abnormality is detected vibration sense is tested more proximally.

Tactile discrimination

Is tested by determining at what distance apart two points of an instrument such as a compass can be distinguished as separate entities. In the fingers this is less than 0.5 cm.

Co-ordination

This can only be accurately assessed in the absence of gross weakness or sensory loss. Co-ordination is assessed by the following techniques.

1. ### Rapid alternating movements

   The patient rapidly supinates and pronates one hand on the dorsum of the other or alternatively a rapid tapping action of the hand is carried out. An abnormality is designated disdiadokokinesis.

2. ### The finger nose test

   The examiner's finger is held approximately two feet from the patient who alternately touches his own nose and the finger of the examiner, first with the eyes open and then with the eyes closed. The examiner's finger can be moved into various positions to increase the difficulty of the manoeuvre.

   Two abnormalities may occur.

   i. *Past pointing.* The patient's finger overshoots either the examiner's finger or his own nose.

   ii. *Intention tremor.* A tremor not present at rest but occurring and increasing in intensity on approaching the finger or the nose. Past pointing and intention tremor frequently occur together.

3. *Rebound*

The examiner attempts to overcome flexion at the elbow by grasping the patient's wrist. If rebound is present, on abruptly releasing the wrist the arm violently flexes and the patient may strike himself in the face unless this is prevented by the examiner's other arm.

EXAMINATION OF THE LOWER LIMB

The same scheme of examination is performed as described under examination of the upper limb. Posture and involuntary movements are noted as is the presence of wasting and/or fasciculation. *Tone* is assessed by supporting the limb at the thigh and foot and putting it through a full range of passive movements. The following methods are used to test *power.*

Dorsiflexion of the foot

The examiner grasps the dorsum of the foot with his right hand and attempts to plantar flex the actively dorsiflexed foot.

Plantar-flexion of the foot

The examiner grasps the plantar surface of the foot and attempts to overcome plantar flexion. It is now convenient to test for *ankle clonus.* The examiner supports the partly flexed knee and abruptly dorsiflexes the relaxed foot, pressure being maintained against the sole. In the presence of clonus oscillating movements of the foot occur which may be sustained or of short duration.

Flexion of the knee

The examiner supports the knee with the left hand and grasps the ankle with the right hand, attempting to overcome knee flexion.

Extension of the knee

The flexed knee is supported by the left arm and the patient extends his knee against resistance supplied by the examiner's right hand at the ankle.

Patellar clonus can now be tested. The extended leg is relaxed while the examiner grasps the upper border of the patella, and with an abrupt movement displaces the patella downwards along the line of the leg, maintaining constant pressure. In the presence of clonus oscillatory movements of the patella occur which may be sustained or of short duration.

Flexion of the hip

The patient lifts the extended leg off the bed thereby flexing the hip. The examiner applies pressure over the lower end of the femur in an attempt to overcome this flexion.

Extension of the hip

The patient forces his extended leg into the bed while the examiner grips the heel and attempts to flex the extended leg.

Reflexes

Knee jerk (L.3.4)

The examiner supports the partially flexed, relaxed legs with his forearm behind the knees. The quadriceps tendon on one side and then the other is struck with the reflex hammer, contraction of the quadriceps and extension of the knee being observed.

Ankle jerk (S.1.)

The patient flexes the knee and rotates the leg outwards, placing his foot on the other tibia. The examiner then dorsiflexes the ankle and while maintaining pressure strikes the Achilles tendon with the reflex hammer. Plantar flexion of the ankle is observed following contraction of the calf muscles.

The reflexes are recorded as before.

Plantar response (S.1.)

A pointed object such as the end of the reflex hammer is stroked from the heel along the lateral border of the sole of the foot and then across the heads of the metatarsals. Initially, gentle stroking is used, but firmer stroking may be required to elicit the plantar response. Normally flexion and drawing together of the toes occurs — the flexor plantar response. With an upper motor neurone lesion dorsiflexion of the big toe occurs, sometimes associated with fanning and extension of the remaining toes — the extensor plantar response. With sensitive feet the sign may be difficult to interpret because of active withdrawal of the leg.

Abdominal reflexes (T.8 – 12)

The patient lies in bed with the abdominal muscles relaxed. The reflexes are elicited on both sides in the upper, mid and lower abdomen by a firm brisk stroke from within outwards with the pointed end of the reflex hammer. Any contraction of the underlying muscle is observed. The reflexes are lost in upper motor neurone lesions affecting that side, or in lower motor neurone lesions of the appropriate segment. Old age, obesity, previous pregnancy and abdominal surgery make the elicitation of the reflexes difficult.

Cremasteric Reflex (L.1)

The skin of the upper inner aspect of the thigh is gently stroked and subsequent contraction of the cremasteric muscle retracts the testicle on that side. The reflex may be lost in upper motor neurone lesions.

Anal Reflex

The skin on either side of the anus is pricked with a pin, normally resulting in brisk contraction of the anus. This reflex is lost in lesions involving the lower sacral nerve roots or cauda equina.

Sensation

The same principles apply as for the upper limb, with light touch, pin prick and temperature being assessed in the same way.

Joint position sense

This is assessed by grasping the sides of the terminal phalanx of the big toe, making small movements of flexion and extension, and asking the patient to indicate in which direction the toe moves. Gross abnormalities of position sense can be demonstrated by asking the patient to point to his foot, which is placed in various positions while his eyes are closed.

Vibration sense

This is assessed by placing the vibrating tuning fork over the malleoli and if absent it is assessed proximally by placing the tuning fork over the tibia, patella, iliac crest, vertebrae and ribs.

Tactile discrimination

This is assessed as in the hand, the minimum difference detectable between the two points on the sole being 4.0 cm.

Co-ordination

Heel-shin test

The patient is asked to place his heel on his opposite knee; intention tremor of the heel may be observed at this point. The heel is then run down the length of the shin to the foot in a smooth movement and any inco-ordination is observed. This is then repeated on the other side.

Rapid alternating movements of the feet

These are tested by asking the patient to tap the examiner's hand with his foot.

Intention tremor

It is tested by asking the patient to touch the examiner's outstretched finger by raising his foot off the bed.

Rhomberg's sign

The patient stands with his heels together and his toes pointing outwards and is then asked to close his eyes. In the normal situation the patient sways slightly with the eyes closed. Cerebellar and posterior column lesions can be differentiated in that any unsteadiness due to a posterior column lesion is accentuated with the eyes closed, while no difference is noted with a cerebellar lesion.

Heel-toe walking

Lesser degrees of ataxia may be detected when the patient walks in a straight line, placing one foot in front of the other, the heel abutting against the toe. Similar differentiation between cerebellar and posterior column lesions can be appreciated with the eyes open and closed.

NEUROLOGICAL DIAGNOSIS

A first stage diagnosis of the site of a neurological lesion is made from the resultant constellation of physical signs. The aetiological diagnosis may not be evident at this stage and requires correlation with the history of the illness, particularly noting the mode of onset or progression. The following are examples.

An upper motor neurone lesion

The features are:

1. *Weakness without wasting*

   The weakness has a characteristic distribution in that in the lower limb it is more marked in the flexors than in the extensors, while in the upper limb it is more marked in the extensors than the flexors. Initially the weakness involves distal and proximal muscles equally while in the recovery stage coarser proximal movements recover earlier than finer movements of the hands and feet.

2. *Increased tone with clonus*

   There is spasticity of the clasp-knife variety, meaning that on attempting to overcome resistance in a limb tone suddenly diminishes. For example, in the lower limb, on attempting to overcome extension the leg suddenly flexes easily. Clonus is only demonstrable in the presence of marked spasticity. Following upper motor neurone lesions tone is often not increased for a period of days to weeks.

3. *Increased deep tendon reflexes*

   Superficial reflexes are absent.

4. *An extensor plantar response*

The commonest example of an upper motor neurone lesion is hemiplegia. The characteristic posture is one of flexion, adduction and pronation in the upper limb and extension of the lower limb. Consequently, on walking the leg is swung outwards and there is dragging of the toe due to plantar flexion of the extended leg.

Causes of a hemiplegia

i. *Vascular*. Haemorrhage, thrombosis or embolus.

   a. *Lesions in the territory of the internal carotid artery* often result in a hemiplegia especially if a large area of the hemisphere or the internal capsule is involved. There may be associated hemi-anaesthesia, aphasia (if the dominant hemisphere is involved) and homonymous hemianopia. Stenosis of the extra-cranial portion of the internal carotid artery may also result in a hemiplegia on the contralateral side associated with a bruit over the stenosis.

b. *Lesions in the territory of the vertebrobasilar artery.* Due to the close proximity of many structures within the confines of the brain stem vascular lesions in this area usually produce bilateral signs. In addition to those of an upper motor neurone lesion, there may be cranial nerve palsies, cerebellar involvement, sensory disturbance and Horner's syndrome.

ii. *Tumours.* In association with the hemiplegia there may be other signs which depend on the site of the tumour. Papilloedema will be present if there is raised intra-cranial pressure.

iii. *Demyelinating Diseases.* The physical signs may indicate more than one lesion.

Lower motor neurone lesion

The features are:

1. **Weakness with wasting**

   The weakness may be more marked peripherally than proximally and involves flexors and extensors equally.

2. **Hypotonia**

3. **Dimished deep tendon reflexes**

   If the reflexes cannot be elicited then they may become demonstrable using reinforcement. To do this the patient is distracted by asking him to attempt to pull his clenched hands apart while the examiner endeavours to elicit the appropriate reflex.

4. **An absent or flexor plantar response**

5. **Trophic changes**

   Occur in long standing lower motor neurone lesions and are manifest by thin, shiny, hairless skin with brittle nails.

Neuropathies are commonly due to lesions of nerve roots, median nerve (carpal tunnel syndrome), ulnar nerve and lateral popliteal nerve. Since the decline in the incidence of poliomyelitis, the commonest polyneuropathy is a peripheral neuropathy which may be associated with distal sensory loss of the glove and stocking type. A peripheral neuropathy may be purely motor or purely sensory, but is commonly mixed.

Causes

i.   Guillian-Barré syndrome
ii. Diabetes
iii. Carcinoma
iv. Nutritional deficiencies (thiamine and vitamin B.12)
v.   Drugs and toxins, including alcohol
vi. Collagen disorders
vii. Miscellaneous, e.g. amyloid
viii. Idiopathic.

Specific nerve lesions due to trauma or pressure occur and are beyond scope of this book. A detailed account of these can be had from "Aids to the Investigation of Peripheral Nerve Injuries" – London, H.M. Stationery Office, War Memorandum 7, 1943.

Myopathy

The features are weakness with wasting, the weakness characteristically being proximal. Weakness of neck flexion occurs early. Deep tendon reflexes will be preserved unless there is gross wasting. Sensation is normal and plantar reflexes are flexor.

Causes

i.   Hereditary muscular dystrophies
ii. Thyrotoxicosis
iii. Carcinoma
iv. Collagen disorders.

Spinal cord compression

While spinal cord compression may produce lower motor neurone signs at the level of the lesion and upper motor neurone signs below the level, the most important clinical sign is the detection of a sensory level. This is demonstrated by examining all modalities of sensation, moving proximally from affected areas. This can most easily be elicited by lightly drawing a pin or wisp of cotton wool over the skin and running proximally, noting when sensation first becomes normal. This procedure is repeated on the opposite side. The actual level of the lesion is usually one or two dermatomes above the sensory level elicited.

Causes

i.   Trauma

ii. Intervertebral disc protrusion

iii. Vertebral collapse (secondary carcinoma)

iv. Tumours such as meningioma and glioma

Other spinal cord lesions are:

v.   Demyelinating disorders

vi. Vascular lesions

vii. Syringomyelia

viii. Vitamin B.12 deficiency (sub-acute combined degeneration of the cord).

Extra-pyramidal diseases

Involuntary movements occur (page 29) associated with hypertonia which involves both flexion and extension and may be either jerky (cog-wheel) or uniform, depending on the presence or absence of tremor. The posture is one of universal flexion with slowness of movement, immobility of the face and excessive salivation. The resultant gait is shuffling and may be festinating, the patient hurrying with small steps with a bent posture as if trying to catch up to his centre of gravity.

Causes

i. Parkinson's disease

ii. Encephalitis

iii. Vascular lesions

iv. Drugs e.g. Phenothiazines

v. Toxins e.g. carbon monoxide

Cerebellar lesions

The features are:

1. *Inco-ordination*
   This is manifest by dysarthia, ataxia of the limbs and gait, disdiadokokinesis, intention tremor, past pointing and rebound.

2. *Hypotonia*

3. *Pendular reflexes*
   To differentiate these from normal reflexes the patient sits on the side of the bed with his feet off the ground. The normal reflex produces a sharp displacement of the limb which returns to its position of rest with little tendency to overshoot that point. With pendular reflexes the leg continues to swing a number of times before coming to rest.

4. *Nystagmus*
   This is phasic in type with the quick component towards the side of the lesion.

5. *Flexor plantar responses*

The signs of cerebellar disease occur on the side of the lesion. Ataxia of the limbs may not be manifest with the patient lying in bed, only becoming evident on getting the patient to walk. The gait is unsteady and on a broad base.

Causes
i.   Hereditary cerebellar ataxias (Friedreich's, etc.)
ii.   Demyelinating disorders
iii. Tumours
         primary
         secondary
         non-metastatic demyelination (especially with carcinoma of the bronchus)
iv.   Toxins – alcohol
v.   Drugs – dilantin
vi.   Vascular lesions
vii. Cerebellar abscess
viii. Myxoedema.

False localising signs

The physical signs produced by an intracranial space occupying lesion usually indicate its site. However, in the presence of raised intracranial pressure there may occur a number of signs which do not necessarily have localising value — false localising signs.

1. Unilateral or bilateral sixth nerve palsy
2. Third nerve palsy
3. Bilateral extensor plantar responses
4. Bilateral grasp reflex
5. Extensor plantar response occurring on the same side as the cerebral space occupying lesion
6. Cerebellar signs occurring with frontal lobe lesions
7. Frontal lobe signs occurring with cerebellar lesions.

THE EXAMINATION OF THE UNCONSCIOUS PATIENT

Any history that can be obtained from other persons concerning the onset of coma should be sought. The setting in which the patient is found is important — such items as empty bottles may provide the important clue to the diagnosis.

The following scheme of examination should be followed.

1. *Colour*

   Evidence of *shock* manifest by a grey appearance, shallow respirations and clamminess of the skin; *cyanosis* consequent on respiratory failure or swallowing of the tongue; *flushed appearance* from carbon monoxide poisoning; *bruising* denoting injury; *bleeding* from anticoagulant drugs or an underlying disorder of coagulation.

2. *Position of the patient*

   Opisthotonos signifies meningeal irritation; abnormal posture of a limb signifies an underlying fracture.

3. *Breathing*

   The deep, rapid breathing of diabetic coma; irregularity of the breathing with Cheyne-Stokes respiration can occur with any cause of deep coma, but in particular is associated with intracranial disturbances.

4. *Dehydration*

This commonly occurs in hyperglycaemic coma, severe infections and uraemia.

Examination of the head

1. *Odour*

Characteristic odours occur with alcohol, diabetes, hepatic coma and uraemia. Even if the odour of alcohol is detected other causes of coma must be excluded.

2. *The tongue*

This may provide further evidence of dehydration and is often bitten in epilepsy.

3. *Palpation of the skull and neck*

Following inspection, the skull is palpated for evidence of haematomas, abrasions and lacerations. Neck rigidity may be evident from the posture of the patient, but is elicited by placing the hand under the occiput and attempting to flex the neck. Neck rigidity is often associated with a positive *Kernig's sign.* This is elicited by flexing the patient's leg at the hip and knee and then attempting to extend the knee. When positive, the knee will not extend more than $90°$. Neck rigidity signifies meningeal irritation due to meningitis or subarachnoid haemorrhage.

4. *Eyes, pupils and fundi*

In the presence of an acute intra-cranial lesion there may be conjugate deviation of the eyes towards the side of the lesion. Unequal pupils may occur with a dilated pupil occurring first on the side of the lesion and indicating raised intra-cranial pressure or a third nerve palsy associated with subarachnoid haemorrhage from an aneurysm of the posterior communicating artery. Bilateral small pupils suggest morphine poisoning or a brain stem haemorrhage. Papilloedema is further evidence of increased intra-cranial pressure. The presence of a typical retinopathy indicates pre-existing diabetes, uraemia or hypertension while a subhyaloid haemorrhage indicates a subarachnoid haemorrhage.

5. *Facial weakness*

This is manifest as facial asymmetry.

6. *Nostrils and ears*

Any bleeding is noted. Draining cerebro-spinal fluid indicates a fracture of the skull. The meatus and drum are inspected for evidence of trauma and infection.

7. *Auscultation of the skull*

This is carried out as described on page 10.

Examination of the limbs

Injection marks suggest diabetes or drug addiction. Tone of the limbs is assessed by raising each limb from the bed and allowing it to fall unsupported. Flaccidity, in association with hemiplegia will be manifest by the limbs on the affected side flopping, whereas the unaffected limbs retain their tone. This flaccidity is usually associated with decrease of the deep tendon reflexes while the plantar response is extensor, although on occasions flaccidity may be associated with exaggerated reflexes. Later, signs of increased tone and hyperreflexia develop on the affected side. While a unilateral extensor plantar response indicates a localised cerebral lesion, bilateral extensor plantar responses may have no localising value as they occur in any form of deep coma and may then be associated with generalised hyporeflexia. Failure to move the limbs on the affected side on painful stimulation may provide the first clue to the presence of hemiplegia.

Examination of the body

A complete physical examination is now carried out. This may reveal causative factors such as evidence of pre-existing hypertension, presence of atrial fibrillation, cardiac murmurs or signs of underlying cirrhosis of the liver.

Examination of the urine

Catheterization of the bladder may be required. The important findings could be:

1. *Sugar and ketone bodies*

   In large amounts they indicate hyperglycaemic coma which should be confirmed either by "Dextrostix" examination of the peripheral blood or measurement of the true blood glucose level. Transient glycosuria may occur with raised intra-cranial pressure while ketones alone may occur with starvation and consequently can occur in any prolonged coma.

2. *Proteinuria*

   If heavy, indicates renal disease and uraemia as the probable cause of coma. Transient proteinuria occurs with raised intracranial pressure. If protein is detected in the urine then microscopic examination should be carried out for cells, casts and organisms.

Examination of the cerebro-spinal fluid

The only indication for lumbar puncture is the presence of meningism, the common causes being subarachnoid haemorrhage and meningo-encephalitis.

Examination of the stomach contents and blood

If a positive diagnosis has not been made, and as drug overdose is such a common cause of coma, it is essential to wash the stomach contents out and have them analysed. Similarly blood samples should be taken for the estimation of levels of barbiturates, alcohol, etc.

Causes of Coma

1. *Drug overdose*

   Barbiturates, carbon monoxide, salicylates, bromides, tranquillisers, anti-depressants and alcohol

2. *Head injuries*

   Cerebral concussion, subdural haematoma, extradural haematoma, brain damage

3. *Sub-arachnoid haemorrhage and intra-cranial vascular lesions*

   Due to haemorrhage, thrombosis or embolism

4. *Diabetes*
Hypoglycaemia or hyperglycaemia

5. *Epilepsy*

6. *Severe infections*
Meningo-encephalitis, cerebral abscess secondary to otitis media, septicaemia

7. *Hysteria*

8. *Rarer causes*
Hepatic coma, respiratory failure, uraemia, adrenal failure, myxoedema, hypercalcaemia and raised intra-cranial pressure, e.g., cerebral tumour.

THE CARDIO-VASCULAR SYSTEM

A systematic examination of the cardiovascular system begins with the pulse.

THE PULSE

The pulse is examined by palpating the right radial artery with the index, middle and ring fingers. The following are determined.
1. Rate
2. Rhythm
3. Pressure and form of the pulse wave
4. State of the vessel wall
5. Comparison of the pulses.

Rate and rhythm

There is a wide variation in the normal rate. The accepted range for an adult in the resting state is 60-90 beats per minute. A regular pulse rate under 60 beats per minute may be due to complete heart block (usually less than 50) or sinus bradycardia and the latter may be associated with:
1. Athletes (physiological)
2. Myxoedema
3. Digitalis
4. Raised intracranial pressure

5. Jaundice.

A rapid regular pulse rate of 90-160 beats per minute (sinus tachycardia) may be associated with:

1. Emotion
2. Exercise
3. Fever
4. Shock
5. Thyrotoxicosis
6. Cardiac failure
7. Drugs such as nicotine, caffeine and amphetamine.

A rapid irregular pulse rate of more than 90 beats per minute, but less than 160 beats per minute, is a cardiac arrhythmia which may be:

1. Atrial fibrillation
2. Extra systoles.

A very rapid pulse rate of more than 160 beats per minute is also indicative of a cardiac arrythmia which may be:

1. Paroxysmal atrial tachycardia
2. Paroxysmal ventricular tachycardia
3. Atrial fibrillation
4. Atrial flutter (commonly 150 beats per minute).

Carotid sinus massage may help to differentiate these conditions. The carotid sinus is located at the bifurcation of the common carotid artery at the upper border of the thyroid cartilage near the angle of the jaw. Carotid sinus massage is carried out with the patient lying flat and the head extended and turned slightly towards the right side. The right carotid sinus is massaged first with either three fingers or the thumb for no more than five seconds, while auscultating over the praecordium. If this does not affect the arrhythmia the left sinus is massaged. Simultaneous bilateral carotid sinus massage is dangerous especially in the elderly and those with cerebral vascular disease.

While no change in the rate may occur, in paroxysmal atrial tachycardia the rate may be restored suddenly to normal; in paroxysmal ventricular tachycardia no change in the rate will occur; in atrial flutter the rate may be slowed abruptly during the period of sinus massage.

Exercise may help in differentiating atrial fibrillation from extra-systoles. In atrial fibrillation the irregularity of the pulse is accentuated by exercise while the irregularity usually diminishes with extrasystoles. Exercise is also used to differentiate sinus bradycardia from heart block. If the pulse rate does not increase on exercise, heart block is probable.

Causes of cardiac arrhythmias

Atrial fibrillation and atrial flutter
i. Hypertensive heart disease
ii. Ischaemic heart disease
iii. Mitral valve disease
iv. Thyrotoxicosis
v. Atrial septal defect
vi. Constrictive pericarditis
vii. Miscellaneous.

Paroxysmal atrial tachycardia
i. Idiopathic
ii. Ischaemic heart disease
iii. Thyrotoxicosis
iv. Digitalis intoxication (with 2 to 1 block).

Paroxysmal ventricular tachycardia
i. Hypertensive heart disease
ii. Ischaemic heart disease
iii. Aortic valve disease
iv. Digitalis intoxication
v. Idiopathic.

Heart block
i. Hypertensive heart disease
ii. Ischaemic heart disease
iii. Digitalis intoxication
iv. Congenital.

The Pressure and Form of the Pulse Wave

An assessment of systolic blood pressure is made by compressing the radial artery with the index finger, palpating the pulse with the middle finger and obliterating the ulnar collateral pulse with the ring finger. The degree of pressure necessary to obliterate the radial pulse gives an estimation of the systolic pressure and this should be confirmed with the sphygmomanometer. The pulse pressure is the difference between the systolic and diastolic pressures. The pulse pressure and duration of the pulse wave determine the form of the pulse which may be:

1. Normal.
2. Small volume. A low pulse pressure of short duration occurring in shock or mitral stenosis.
3. Plateau pulse. A low pulse pressure of long duration occurring in aortic stenosis.
4. Large volume pulse. A large pulse pressure of normal duration occurring in hypertension.
5. Collapsing pulse. A large pulse pressure of short duration occurring in aortic incompetence and high output states including anaemia, patent ductus arteriosus, and fever. The abrupt, briefly sustained rise of the collapsing pulse is accentuated by elevating the arm and palpating the radial artery with the palmar surface of the hand. A collapsing pulse is associated with easily visible carotid pulsations (Corrigan's sign). Capillary pulsation may be seen in the nail bed on application of gentle pressure to the tip of the nail.

Other types of pulse are described — dicrotic, bisferiens and anacrotic — but these are rarely of clinical value.

State of the vessel wall

This is assessed by obliterating the radial pulse and feeling the vessel wall. In young people this is normally not palpable while in the presence of arterial disease a thickened vessel wall may be palpable.

Comparison of the pulses

The form of the pulse wave is compared in both radial arteries and a common abnormality is absence or diminution in pulse pressure in one radial artery. This may be due to:

1. Previous arterial catheterisation
2. Congenital absence of one radial artery
3. Dissection of the aorta
4. Embolus.

The peripheral pulses are then palpated. The posterior tibial artery is felt behind the medial malleolus and the dorsalis pedis is palpated between the heads of the first and second metatarsal bones. If these pulses are abnormal then the popliteal artery should be palpated, but may be difficult to feel and requires firm palpation in the popliteal fossa. The femoral pulses are palpated just below the inguinal ligament. The brachial artery is palpated just to the medial side of the biceps tendon and the axillary artery is palpated by firm pressure against the neck of the humerus.

DETERMINATION OF THE BLOOD PRESSURE

The patient should be relaxed with the right arm uncovered to the shoulder. The sphygmomanometer cuff is applied to the middle of the upper arm and then inflated until the radial pulse disappears. This reading indicates the approximate systolic pressure. After deflation the cuff is reinflated to a pressure of 30 mm mercury above the systolic pressure obtained by palpation, the stethoscope being applied lightly over the brachial artery. Auscultation is conducted during slow deflation of the cuff and when sounds are first heard this represents systolic pressure. Diastolic pressure is the point at which the sounds disappear.

A casual reading of the blood pressure may not be a true guide to the presence or absence of meaningful hypertension as both the systolic and diastolic pressures can be elevated by emotion. Elevation of the systolic pressure with a normal diastolic pressure is commonly found in elderly patients with atherosclerosis.

While there are no strict criteria for the definition of hypertension a blood pressure reading of 150/95 should be viewed with suspicion. Hypertension may be either transient or sustained.

Transient

1. Emotion
2. Acute glomerulo-nephritis
3. Phaeochromocytoma
4. Toxaemia of pregnancy.

Sustained

1. Essential
2. Renal disease
      chronic pyelonephritis
      chronic glomerulo-nephritis
      renal artery stenosis
      polycystic kidneys
3. Co-arctation of the aorta
4. Endocrine disorders
      Cushing's disease
      thyrotoxicosis
      phaeochromocytoma
      primary aldosteronism.

In sustained hypertension left ventricular hypertrophy, hypertensive retinopathy and proteinuria are important in assessing the duration and degree of the hypertension.

THE EXAMINATION OF THE PULSATIONS IN THE NECK

Pulsations in the neck may be venous or arterial and are sometimes difficult to differentiate. As a general rule, if a pulsation is more easily seen than felt, it is venous; while in contrast arterial pulsation is more readily felt than seen. A venous pulse will rise during expiration, coughing or straining and compression of the upper abdomen, while it will fall if the patient sits up. These manoeuvres will not affect arterial pulsation. Arterial pulsation is commonly seen in the normal patient, but if prominent is suggestive of aortic incompetence.

Estimation of central venous pressure

To estimate central venous pressure the jugular veins are inspected with the patient reclining at an angle of 45°. In normal subjects the venous pulse is not visible. If the venous pressure is elevated the distended external and internal jugular veins may be visible. The rise in central venous pressure is estimated by taking zero pressure at the horizontal line drawn to meet the junction of the manubrium and the body of the sternum. If there is doubt about the elevation of the venous pressure compression over the upper abdomen may cause the venous pressure to rise and thus become more easily visible. On releasing the abdominal compression the level of pulsation falls. This manoeuvre may not be successful because the internal jugular veins may be obscured in obese patients. The external jugular vein should then be examined by applying a finger above the mid point of the clavicle, producing filling of the vein. When the finger is removed the column of blood falls to the level corresponding to central venous pressure. Care must be taken in the interpretation of any elevation of the external jugular pressure as this vein may be compressed by the cervical fascia and thus may not represent true central venous pressure. In such a situation venous pulsation is absent and the pressure may fall on movement of the neck.

In addition to the differentiating features described, the venous pulse is also characterised by two distinct waves in each cycle producing a "double flicker". It is important to realise that if the central venous pressure is markedly raised no such pulsations may be visible in the neck until the patient is examined sitting upright.

Variations in the form of the venous pulse occur, but their interpretation is difficult. Identification of the "a" and "v" waves is assisted by simultaneous palpation of the opposite carotid artery.

Examples are:

1. Absent "a" waves in atrial fibrillation resulting in a single forceful venous wave.
2. Giant "v" waves resulting in a similar forceful venous wave of greater amplitude occurring in tricuspid incompetence.

3. Giant "a" waves are conspicuous in tricuspid stenosis, but may occur in any condition associated with powerful right ventricular contraction, e.g., pulmonary stenosis, pulmonary hypertension.
4. Similar large "a" waves occur in complete heart block and are designated cannon waves. They differ from the usual "a" wave in that they occur irregularly.

Causes of a raised venous pressure

While very slow heart rates and increased blood volume can result in increased venous pressure the important causes are:

i. Right ventricular failure
ii. Tricuspid incompetence
iii. Superior vena caval obstruction
iv. Constrictive pericarditis and pericardial effusion.

EXAMINATION OF THE PRAECORDIUM

Inspection

The aims of inspection are:

1. *To determine the position of the apex beat*

   It is the lowest and outermost point of cardiac pulsation and is usually found in the fifth left intercostal space internal to the mid-clavicular line. This is the line drawn perpendicularly from the mid-point of the clavicle. It should be emphasised that the nipple line is not necessarily the mid-clavicular line. Intercostal spaces are determined following identification of the second costal cartilage and are numbered according to the number of the costal cartilage above. The position of the apex beat may be altered by skeletal deformities and may not be visible in people with a thick chest wall, obesity or emphysema.

2. *To detect the presence of right ventricular enlargement*

   While this is best appreciated by palpation it may be evident as a visible pulsation at the left sternal edge associated with a marked epigastric pulsation which needs to be differentiated from aortic pulsation.

Fig. 1a, 1b, 1c & 1d. The Normal and Abnormal Forms of the Jugular Venous Pulse

Two distinct pulsations may be seen in each cardiac cycle. The first or "a" wave precedes the carotid pulse and is due to contraction of the right atrium. This is followed by the "x" descent due to atrial relaxation and this may be interrupted by an inconspicuous wave, the "c" wave. The second, or "v" wave, follows the carotid pulse and is due to the gradual filling of the right atrium while the tricuspid valve is closed. This is followed by the "y" descent which represents ventricular filling. The clinical differentiation of the component venous waves is difficult, especially if the heart rate is rapid or if the venous pressure is considerably elevated. Simultaneous palpation of the opposite carotid artery will assist in timing the "a" and "v" waves.

1a Normal venous waves
1b Carotid pulsation
1c Giant "a" waves
1d Giant "v" waves

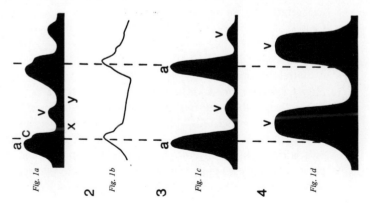

Fig. 1a

Fig. 1b

Fig. 1c

Fig. 1d

3. *To detect other vascular abnormalities*
   i. Pulsation in the right or left upper chest due to an aneurysm of the ascending aorta.
   ii. Arterial pulsation seen over the lower borders of the scapulae indicating the presence of collateral arterial circulation associated with co-arctation of the aorta. This is best seen with the patient leaning forward on his folded arms.
   iii. Abnormally distended veins associated with inferior or superior vena-caval obstruction.

Palpation

The aims of palpation are to confirm the findings of inspection and:
1. *To localise the apex beat and to determine its form*
   The palm of the hand should be lightly placed over the apex beat with the fingers pointing towards the axilla. More accurate localisation is possible by light palpation with the finger tips. The apex beat may be neither visible nor palpable where there is a thick chest wall, obesity, emphysema or abnormalities of the pericardium such as an effusion or constrictive pericarditis.

   The form of the apex beat may be:
   i. *Normal*
   ii. *Left ventricular.* A localised heaving impulse which is an exaggeration of the norm.
      Causes
      a. hypertension
      b. aortic valve disease
      c. mitral incompetence.
   iii. *Right ventricular.* A diffuse impulse which has a tapping rather than a thrusting quality. A right ventricular apex beat is frequently associated with right ventricular enlargement which is manifest as a heaving along the left sternal edge associated with prominent pulsation in the epigastrium. A parasternal heave is a more reliable indication of right ventricular enlargment than a tapping apex beat.

Causes
a. mitral stenosis
b. other causes of pulmonary hypertension such as chronic obstructive airways disease
c. atrial septal defect
d. pulmonary stenosis.

2. *To detect thrills*

A thrill is a fine palpable vibration accompanying an underlying murmur and signifying the organic nature of that murmur. Light palpation with the palmar surfaces of the fingers is essential and correct positioning of the patient is necessary (see appropriate valve lesions).

Percussion

If the apex beat is impalpable percussion is useful to determine the left border of the heart and is carried out by percussing along the fifth intercostal space from the axilla.

Auscultation

Auscultation is carried out in the following four areas which however do not represent the anatomical positions of the valves.
1. The mitral area situated at the cardiac apex
2. The tricuspid area at the lower left sternal edge
3. The aortic area in the second right intercostal space close to the sternum
4. The pulmonary area in the second left intercostal space close to the sternum.

The aims of auscultation are to determine the character of the heart sounds and to detect the presence of cardiac murmurs.

1. *Heart sounds*

Determine if both heart sounds are clearly audible in all areas and note which sound is the loudest. The second heart sound is normally louder in the aortic and pulmonary areas while the first sound is louder in the tricuspid and mitral areas. Third and fourth sounds, often difficult to distinguish, may be audible and best heard internal to the apex beat. In children and adolescents the third heart sound is usually physiological while in adult life the additional sound signifies heart failure.

Abnormalities

a. A loud first heart sound at the apex. This may accompany any tachycardia, but should alert the physician to the possibility of underlying mitral stenosis.

b. A loud second sound at the aortic area. This is associated with systemic hypertension or an aneurysm of the ascending aorta.

c. A loud second heart sound in the pulmonary area is associated with pulmonary hypertension.

d. Accentuation of the normal splitting of the second heart sound in the pulmonary area. The pulmonary second sound is normally split, having an early aortic and later pulmonary component. The split increases during inspiration owing to prolongation of systole due to the increased venous return to the heart. Accentuation of the pulmonary component occurs in association with pulmonary hypertension. Fixed splitting, that is failure of the splitting to vary with respiration, occurs with an atrial septal defect.

Other variations such as reversed splitting of the second sound, splitting of the first heart sound and systolic clicks are described.

e. Gallop rhythm. This is a triple rhythm having a cadence resembling that of a galloping horse. In general, the extra sound is best heard internal to the apex beat in left ventricular failure and at the lower left sternal edge in right ventricular failure. It occurs only when the heart rate is more than 100 beats per minute. If the extra sound is due to a third heart sound the gallop rhythm is called proto-diastolic; if it is due to a fourth heart sound it is called pre-systolic. However, as the ventricular rate is fast the differentiation is difficult. If the two sounds are superimposed the rhythm is called a summation gallop. The importance of a triple rhythm due to the third sound is that it is evidence of ventricular failure; the disappearance of the triple rhythm signifies improvement in cardiac function. Its persistence is a bad prognostic sign.

2. *Cardiac murmurs*

These are produced by turbulence of blood flow and in order to localise their site of production the following criteria are determined.

i. Timing – systolic or diastolic
ii. Point of maximum intensity
iii. Radiation
iv. Presence of a thrill.

Cardiac murmurs may be designated as:

Pansystolic. A blowing sound heard during systole beginning at or shortly after the first heart sound and continuing throughout systole up to or even obliterating the second sound. A pansystolic murmur arises from the mitral valve, tricuspid valve or is associated with a ventricular septal defect.

Midsystolic. A harsher sound in systole commencing shortly after the first heart sound and terminating before the second sound, reaching a crescendo in midsystole. Midsystolic murmurs usually arise from the aortic and pulmonary valves, but may also arise from the mitral and tricuspid valves.

Early diastolic. A soft high-pitched sound beginning immediately after the second heart sound and diminishing in intensity during diastole. It is best heard with the diaphragm of the stethoscope. An early diastolic murmur arises from the aortic or pulmonary valve.

Mid-diastolic. A low-pitched rumbling sound heard in mid-diastole which may be associated with presystolic accentuation, the murmur increasing in intensity in late diastole. Presystolic accentuation is not heard with atrial fibrillation. A mid-diastolic murmur is best heard with the bell of the stethoscope and arises from the mitral or tricuspid valve.

CARDIAC LESIONS

Valvular lesions of the heart are each associated with a characteristic murmur and the diagnosis of a particular valvular lesion in the absence of that murmur should be made with caution. Other physical signs often support the diagnosis. The following are the physical signs associated with common valvular lesions.

Acquired valvular lesions

Mitral stenosis

The murmur is mid-diastolic, best heard just internal to the apex beat, and may be associated with a thrill. It is localised and does not radiate. The murmur is accentuated by lying the patient in the left lateral position after increasing the heart rate with exercise. The following physical signs may accompany the murmur.

i.   A loud first heart sound at the mitral area.

ii. An opening snap — a clicking sound immediately preceding the murmur and often loudest internal to the apex beat.

iii. A right ventricular apex beat and/or a parasternal heave. In mitral stenosis the apex beat is not displaced.

iv. An accentuated pulmonary second sound indicating pulmonary hypertension.

v.   A normal or small volume pulse.

vi. Atrial fibrillation is common.

vii. Mitral facies — a flushed appearance over the malar bones.

   Causes

   a. Rheumatic heart disease

   b. D.L.E. (rare)

   c. Atrial myxoma (rare).

Mitral incompetence

The murmur is classically pansystolic, best heard in the mitral area and conducted to the axilla and/or the left sternal edge. However the murmur may occupy only part of systole. It is commonly associated with a thrill. The following physical signs may accompany the murmur.

i. A left ventricular apex beat signifying left ventricular enlargement.
ii. The pulse may be normal or have a collapsing quality.
iii. Atrial fibrillation.

Causes

a. Valvular
rheumatic heart disease
bacterial endocarditis.

b. Functional
secondary to dilatation of the valve ring which may occur with any cause of marked left ventricular enlargement.

c. Sub-valvular
papillary muscle dysfunction commonly associated with myocardial infaction.

Aortic stenosis

The murmur is mid-systolic and of maximum intensity in the aortic area. It is conducted into the neck. In some cases the murmur in fact may be best heard down the left sternal edge or at the apex. An identical murmur may occur in the presence of atheromatous roughening of the aortic valve without significant stenosis (aortic sclerosis).

The following physical signs may accompany the murmur.

i. Plateau pulse
ii. Left ventricular apex beat denoting left ventricular enlargement.

Causes

a. Congenital
bicuspid valve
hypertrophic sub-aortic stenosis

b. Acquired
rheumatic heart disease
aortic sclerosis.

Aortic incompetence

The murmur is early diastolic and heard in the aortic area. It is conducted down the left sternal edge where in fact it may be heard best. The murmur is accentuated by the patient sitting up, leaning forward and holding the breath in expiration. The following physical signs may accompany the murmur.

i. Collapsing pulse
ii. Easily visible carotid pulsations (Corrigan's sign)
iii. Left ventricular apex beat denoting left ventricular enlargement
iv. Capillary pulsation in the nail bed observed by depressing the tip of the nail to partially occlude the underlying circulation
v. Pistol shot sounds over the femoral arteries which may be accompanied by a diastolic murmur (Duroziez's sign).

Causes
a. Congenital
   bicuspid valve
b. Acquired
   rheumatic heart disease
   syphilitic aortitis
   dissecting aneurysm
   severe systemic hypertension
   bacterial endocarditis
   Marfan's syndrome
   collagen diseases.

Tricuspid incompetence

The murmur is soft, pansystolic and of maximum intensity in the tricuspid area, being accentuated by inspiration. This murmur is the exception to the general rule, in that it is not the cardinal sign. The murmur is often difficult to hear either because the valve ring is very large and turbulence may not be produced by the regurgitant stream or because of the frequent association of mitral stenosis and mitral incompetence. The diagnostic accompanying physical signs are:
i. A raised jugular venous pressure with prominent "v" waves
ii. Expansile pulsation of the liver.

These signs are usually accompanied by those of right heart failure and atrial fibrillation.

Causes
a. *Functional.* Implies that there is dilatation of the valve ring secondary to cardiac dilatation, the valve cusps being normal. Cardiac dilatation occurs with cardiac failure and the signs of

tricuspid incompetence disappear if the cardiac size diminishes with treatment.

b. *Rheumatic heart disease.*

c. *Carcinoid syndrome.*

Pulmonary incompetence secondary to pulmonary hypertension

The characteristic murmur is early diastolic and of maximum intensity at the pulmonary area, being conducted down the left sternal edge. The associated physical signs are those of pulmonary hypertension.

i. An accentuated pulmonary second sound which may be widely split
ii. A parasternal heave, denoting right ventricular enlargement
iii. A soft mid-systolic murmur in the pulmonary area
iv. A gallop rhythm at the left sternal edge.

Superimposed on these physical signs may be those of the underlying cause of the pulmonary hypertension — cor pulmonale, mitral stenosis, atrial septal defect, patent ductus arteriosus and pulmonary embolus.

Combined valvular lesions

Mitral stenosis and mitral incompetence

Both characteristic murmurs are present and an assessment of which particular valve lesion is dominant is difficult.

However, a left ventricular type of apex beat favours mitral incompetence while a right ventricular apex beat favours mitral stenosis.

Pulmonary hypertension may complicate mitral valve disease and lead to right ventricular enlargement with functional tricuspid incompetence. Atrial fibrillation is then invariable.

Aortic stenosis and aortic incompetence

Both characteristic murmurs will be present. The pulse gives the clue to the dominant lesion. A plateau pulse signifies aortic stenosis whereas a collapsing pulse signifies aortic incompetence. Pulsus bisferiens, a large volume pulse with a notch on the upstroke, may be present when stenosis and incompetence are of equal and marked severity.

Congenital heart disease

Coarctation of the aorta

This is manifest by hypertension in the upper limbs with relative hypotension in the lower limbs, associated with delayed and diminished femoral pulsations, there being no diagnostic murmur. The following physical signs may be present.

i. A collateral arterial circulation develops over the scapulae and lower ribs. It is best identified with the patient folding his arms and leaning forward and may be associated with a systolic bruit.

ii. A mid-systolic murmur heard in the second left intercostal space close to the sternum, and radiating along the course of the internal mammary arteries.

iii. The murmur of aortic incompetence or stenosis due to either the presence of a bicuspid aortic valve or aneurysmal dilatation of the ascending aorta resulting in dilatation of the aortic ring.

iv. Left ventricular enlargement.

v. An expansile pulsation in the right side of the neck or suprasternal notch due to dilatation of the carotid artery.

Associated conditions

a. Aneurysm of the circle of Willis

b. Bicuspid aortic valve

c. Aneurysmal dilatation of the ascending aorta

d. Bacterial endocarditis

e. Other congenital lesions — patent ductus arteriosus, ventricular septal defect and aortic or subaortic stenosis

f. Turner's syndrome.

Atrial septal defect

There is a left to right shunt and the right ventricular output is two or three times greater than the left ventricular output.

The characteristic physical signs are:

i. A soft mid-systolic murmur in the pulmonary area. There is usually no thrill but the pulmonary artery pulsation may be palpable

ii. Fixed splitting of the second sound in the pulmonary area

iii. A right parasternal heave and a tapping apex beat signifying right ventricular enlargement

iv. Atrial fibrillation or flutter
v. A blowing early diastolic murmur at the left sternal edge due to functional pulmonary incompetence secondary to pulmonary hypertension.

The basal systolic and early diastolic murmurs may be confused with those of aortic stenosis and incompetence unless due regard is paid to the signs associated with right ventricular enlargement. Bacterial endocarditis is rare in atrial septal defect.

Ventricular septal defect

The characteristic murmur is pansystolic, associated with a thrill, and of maximum intensity in the third and fourth intercostal spaces at the left sternal edge.

A heaving apex beat due to left ventricular enlargement often accompanies the murmur.

Bacterial endocarditis occurs commonly, producing emboli to the pulmonary rather than to the systemic circulation.

Patent ductus arteriosus

The characteristic murmur is a "machinery murmur" which is a continuous rumbling murmur occupying the whole of systole and diastole and often associated with a thrill. Systolic accentuation occurs just before the second heart sound. The murmur is best heard in the first or second left intercostal space, the important feature being that it is localised and of maximal intensity lateral to the pulmonary area. The following physical signs may accompany the murmur.

i. A collapsing pulse
ii. A heaving apex beat denoting left ventricular enlargement
iii. A loud pulmonary second sound which may be masked by the murmur.

Bacterial endocarditis occurs commonly with a patent ductus arteriosus.

Pulmonary stenosis

The murmur is mid-systolic, often associated with a thrill and heard best in the pulmonary area. The following physical signs may accompany the murmur.

i. A parasternal heave and tapping apex beat denoting right ventricular enlargement

ii. A prominent "a" wave in the jugular venous pulse.

Dextrocardia

The apex beat is found to the right of the sternum. This may, however, be due to a large pleural effusion or pneumothorax on the left, or collapse of the right lower lobe. However, a congenital form occurs often associated with transposition of the viscera (situs inversus), and may be associated with basal bronchiectasis and malformation of the frontal sinuses.

Tetralogy of Fallot

This is the commonest form of cyanotic congenital heart disease and comprises stenosis of the outflow tract of the right ventricle and/or the pulmonary valve, dextro-position of aorta (overriding aorta), right ventricular enlargement and a ventricular septal defect. The characteristic physical signs are:

i. Central cyanosis

ii. Clubbing

iii. A systolic murmur heard at the left sternal edge between the second to fourth intercostal spaces and frequently accompanied by a thrill.

Other cyanotic congenital heart conditions occur, but their clinical differentiation is difficult.

Having determined the cardiac lesion, the presence or absence of cardiac failure and endocarditis should be established.

SIGNS OF CARDIAC FAILURE

Left ventricular failure

1. Bilateral basal crepitations
2. A gallop rhythm best heard just internal to the apex beat
3. Tachycardia
4. Tachypnoea
5. Pleural effusion

6. Pulsus alternans — a regular rhythm with alternately strong and weak beats — a grave prognostic sign.

Causes
i. Hypertension
ii. Myocardial infarction
iii. Aortic valve lesions
iv. Mitral incompetence.

Right ventricular failure
1. Raised jugular venous pressure
2. Peripheral oedema
3. Hepatic enlargement
4. Ascites.

Causes
i. Secondary to left ventricular failure
ii. Pulmonary heart disease
iii. Congenital heart disease with right ventricular overload
iv. Ischaemic heart disease.

Oedema first appears in the lower legs and is pitting. Firm pressure with the thumb for five to ten seconds will leave a depression which is slow to disappear. The oedema may extend proximally involving the abdomen and thorax. In the recumbent posture it may only be apparent over the sacrum.

Both right and left ventricular failure may occur at the same time, except when due to primary respiratory conditions.

SIGNS OF BACTERIAL ENDOCARDITIS

The following signs, when accompanied by a cardiac murmur and especially if the character of that murmur alters over a period of hours, days or weeks, are suggestive of bacterial endocarditis
1. Low grade fever

2. Emboli
   Linear haemorrhages beneath the nails (splinter haemorrhages)
   Small, red, tender, raised, localised lesions usually occurring on
   the palms of the hands or soles of the feet (Osler's nodes).
   Emboli to larger vessels
   cerebral
   renal
   peripheral
3. Haematuria, which is usually microscopic and due to emboli or an
   associated nephritis
4. Anaemia
5. Splenomegaly
6. Clubbing of the fingers.

PERICARDIAL LESIONS

Uncommon though important cardiac lesions are those involving the
pericardium.

Pericarditis

The cardinal physical sign is a friction rub — a creaking or scratching
sound usually heard best in a localised area at the left sternal edge and
present during systole and diastole.

Causes

i.   Myocardial infarction
ii. Active rheumatic carditis
iii. Collagen diseases
iv. Infections — viral
                   pyogenic
v.   Uraemia
vi. Malignancy.

Pericardial effusion

1. A pericardial friction rub is common.
2. Faint heart sounds with a barely palpable or impalpable apex beat.

3. Generalised cardiac enlargement detected by percussion, but best demonstrated radiologically.
4. Raised central venous pressure due to cardiac tamponade.
   Causes
   Any of the causes of pericarditis may produce an effusion; however, it is rare in myocardial infarction and uraemia.

Constrictive pericarditis

1. Engorged cervical veins which do not pulsate, due to superior vena caval obstruction
2. Hepatic enlargement, ascites and oedema, due to inferior vena caval obstruction
3. Atrial fibrillation occurs commonly
4. Pulsus paradoxus — the pulse is of small volume and the pulse pressure diminishes on inspiration.
   Causes
   a. Tuberculosis
   b. Idiopathic.

THE GASTROINTESTINAL SYSTEM

Examination commences with inspection of the lips and oral cavity.

Examination of the lips

The following abnormalities may occur

Cyanosis (page 2)

Angular stomatitis

Cracks in the skin at the corners of the mouth often associated with local infection. The commonest cause is ill-fitting false teeth, but it also occurs with iron deficiency and other nutritional disorders including vitamin B.12 deficiency.

Leukoplakia

Indurated, greyish-white plaques occurring on the lower lip and commonly a precursor of carcinoma.

Ulceration

Chronic ulceration should be regarded as carcinoma until proved otherwise.

Hereditary haemorrhagic telangiectasia

Multiple telangiectasia occurring predominantly on the lips and surrounding skin and in the oral cavity.

Localised pigmentation (Peutz-Jegher syndrome)

Discrete, brown-black, pigmented spots occurring on and around the lips, associated with small intestinal polyposis.

Herpes simplex
Shallow, acute, painful ulcerations on the outer surface of the lips, often recurrent and often associated with hyperpyrexia.

Examination of the teeth, gums and buccal mucosa
An assessment should be made of the general state of the teeth. If false teeth are present they should be removed so that an adequate inspection of the oral cavity can be made.

The following abnormalities may occur.
Gingivitis
Manifest as redness, swelling and perhaps bleeding around the tooth sockets, being localised or generalised and primary (Vincent's angina) or secondary to an underlying disorder such as a blood dyscrasia.
Bleeding
May be associated with a bleeding tendency such as occurs in scurvy, thrombocytopenia, leukaemia and uraemia.
Hypertrophy
Due to dilantin toxicity or leukaemic infiltration, especially monocytic leukaemia.
Pigmentation
A greyish-black discolouration on the gums occurring in heavy metal poisoning (e.g. bismuth and lead). Pigmentation of the buccal mucosa occurs in conditions such as Addison's disease and haemochromatosis and may be localised opposite the lower second and third molar teeth.
Moniliasis
Small white plaques that can be removed only with difficulty, and seen in association with faulty oral hygiene, leukaemia, broad spectrum antibiotic or steroid therapy.

Examination of the tongue
While a dry tongue occurs in dehydration it is commonly due to mouth breathing. Furring and fissuring of the tongue can occur in health and disease and are of little diagnostic value. Common abnormalities are:

Atrophic glossitis
A smooth red tongue which is often painful, associated with deficiencies of iron, vitamin B.12 or folic acid.

Magenta tongue
Occurring in nutritional deficiencies.

Macroglossia
Associated with acromegaly, amyloid disease, hypothyroidism and mongolism.

Wasting
Occurs in lower motor neurone lesions of the hypoglossal nerve. If bilateral and associated with fibrillation, motor neurone disease is suggested.

Leukoplakia
As with leukoplakia of the lip this is a common precursor of carcinoma of the tongue.

Ulceration
If chronic, carcinoma is likely.

THE ABDOMEN
For descriptive purposes the abdomen is divided into 9 areas by drawing two horizontal lines, one at the level of the lower costal margins and the other between both anterior superior iliac crests. The two vertical lines are extensions of the mid-clavicular lines. (Figure 2)

The areas are designated:
1. Right hypochondrium
2. Epigastrium
3. Left hypochondrium
4. Right lumbar region
5. Umbilical region
6. Left lumbar region
7. Right iliac fossa
8. Hypogastrium
9. Left iliac fossa.

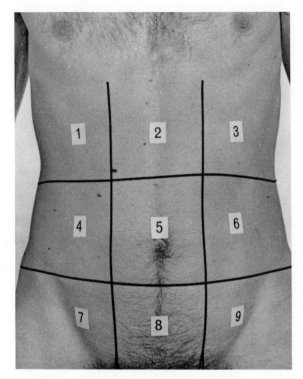

Fig. 2

The abdomen is examined with the patient lying comfortably, hands by his sides and head on one pillow, the bladder ideally having been emptied.

Inspection

The following are noted.

1. *Scars*

   Indicating previous surgery.

2. *Local swellings*

   Such as a hernia or an enlargement of an abdominal or pelvic viscus.

3. *Generalised distension*

Often best appreciated from the foot of the bed and may be due to:

i. fluid (ascites), the distension being predominantly in flanks and often associated with an umbilical hernia

ii. fat

iii. Flatus and faeces

iv. Uterine and ovarian swellings, where the distension appears to arise out of the pelvis.

Physical signs of ascites. In the obese patient the clinical recognition of ascites can be difficult. Ascitic distension may be limited to the flanks or generalised and associated with an umbilical hernia. There is dullness to percussion in both flanks and the dullness shifts on posturing the patient.

To detect ascites percussion is carried out from the umbilicus towards first the left flank and then the right. The note becomes dull in the normal patient in the mid axillary line, while in the presence of ascites dullness to percussion will be found anterior to this line on both sides. The point where dullness is encountered on the left is either marked, or the hand is left on the abdomen while the patient rolls towards the examiner. In the presence of ascites the percussion note at this point becomes resonant (shifting dullness). A similar manoeuvre can be carried out on the right side. Percussion must be carried out below the lower limit of any enlarged viscus such as the liver or spleen. *A fluid thrill* may be detected in the presence of ascites, but is rarely present in the absence of shifting dullness. It is elicited by placing the left hand over the left lateral abdominal wall of the patient and flicking the right lateral abdominal wall. In the presence of ascites or fat a thrill will be felt by the left hand. To prevent the thrill being transmitted through fat the patient places the edge of his hand along the linea alba.

Causes

a. Cirrhosis of the liver

b. Malignancy

c. Congestive cardiac failure

d. Nephrotic syndrome
e. Malabsorption
f. Hepatic vein occlusion
g. Peritoneal infection.

Provided the ascites is not tense, enlarged underlying organs are felt by *ballotment.* This is carried out by placing the right hand on the patient's abdomen with the fingers together and making a sudden flexion movement at the metocarpo-phalangeal joints, thereby displacing fluid and palpating the underlying organ.

4. *Engorged veins*

In the presence of distension or rapid weight loss normal veins may be seen and need to be distinguished from the distended veins occurring in:

  i. *Inferior vena caval obstruction.* The veins are prominent in the flanks and the direction of blood flow is from below upwards.
 ii. *Portal venous hypertension.* The veins may be prominent around the umbilicus (caput medusae) and the direction of flow of blood is away from the umbilicus.

To assess the direction of venous blood flow both index fingers are placed together over an engorged vein. The fingers are then moved apart, thereby emptying the vein. The direction of the blood flow is ascertained by removing each finger alternately and observing subsequent filling of the vein.

5. *Nodules*

Located in or under the skin and may be associated with:

  i. *Metastatic carcinoma.* Usually bronchial; occurring in the scar following surgery for abdominal malignancy; or associated with melanoma.
 ii. *Leukaemia.*
iii. *Campbell de Morgan spots.* Small, bright red, elevated angiomata which do not blanch on pressure and are of no clinical significance.

6. *Intestinal movements*

Writhing movements often associated with borborygmi and observed in intestinal obstruction, pyloric stenosis and incisional herniae.

Palpation

The examiner sits on the right side of the patient who lies comfortably with his head on one pillow and both hands by his sides. It is rarely necessary for the patient to draw up his legs as this in fact does little to relax the abdominal muscles.

Superficial palpation

The examiner's previously warmed hand is placed on the abdominal wall with the fingers together. Gentle flexion movements of the fingers at the metacarpo-phalangeal joints are made commencing at the left iliac fossa and moving in a clockwise direction around the abdomen. Superficial palpation may reveal:

i. Tenderness
ii. Guarding or rigidity of the abdominal muscles suggesting underlying peritoneal irritation
iii. The outline of an enlarged viscus or a tumour
iv. Incisional herniae and divarication of the recti.

Whilst superficial palpation usually reveals no abnormalities it should not be omitted as it helps the examiner to gain the patient's confidence thereby ensuring muscular relaxation for deeper palpation.

To ensure that any mass felt is within the abdominal cavity and not in the abdominal wall the patient's abdominal musculature is contracted by asking him to flex his neck against resistance by the examiner. Intra-abdominal masses become less easily palpable.

Deep palpation

This is carried out in the same manner as with superficial palpation except the movements of the fingers are deeper. Following deep palpation in all areas specific examination is made to detect enlargement of intra-abdominal viscera.

Palpation of the liver (Surface markings, Figure 3)

Palpation commences in the right iliac fossa lateral to the rectus

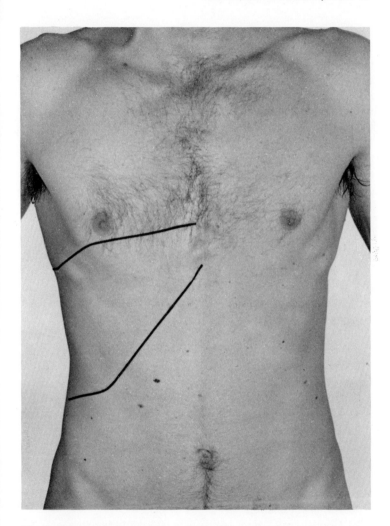

Fig. 3 The surface markings of the liver. The lower border is at the level of the costal margin while the upper border is in the 4th to 5th intercostal space.

muscle with the fingers parallel to the subcostal margin. The patient breathes slowly and deeply through the open mouth. The examiner's hand is advanced towards the subcostal margin in increments of approximately 1 cm during expiration, the hand being kept still during inspiration. Once the liver edge is felt its lower border is outlined and this is later confirmed by percussion. The lower edge may extend into the left hypochondrium and be confused with an enlarged spleen.

It is essential to delineate by percussion the upper border of the liver by percussing downwards in the right mid-clavicular line. The upper border is normally in the fourth right intercostal space or underneath the fifth rib. The following features of an enlarged liver are noted.

i. Size
ii. Tender or non-tender
iii. The character of the lower border, regular or irregular and whether soft or hard.
iv. The character of the surface: smooth or nodular, soft or hard
v. Pulsation. This is elicited by bimanual palpation, the left hand being placed under the patient and the right hand gently on the surface of the enlarged liver. Pulsation may be transmitted from the underlying aorta or occur with tricuspid incompetence, hepatoma and vascular anomalies.

Causes of an enlarged liver
i. *Massive (below the level of the umbilicus)*
   a. Metastatic carcinoma
   b. Right ventricular failure
   c. Alcoholic liver disease
   d. Cirrhosis of the liver complicated by a hepatoma.
ii. *Moderate*
   a. The above causes
   b. Haemochromatosis
   c. Haematological disorders, such as leukaemia, lymphomas
   d. Extra-hepatic cholestasis
   e. Hepatitis — the characteristic feature being tenderness rather than enlargement

   f. Hydatid disease.
iii. *Irregular*
   a. Cirrhosis of the liver especially when complicated by a hepatoma
   b. Metastatic liver disease
   c. Hydatid disease.
iv. *Tender*
   a. Hepatitis due to any cause
   b. Rapid enlargement of the liver, such as occurs in right ventricular failure or malignancy
   c. Hepatoma.

Palpation of the Gall bladder

A distended gall bladder, if palpable, is felt at the junction of the subcostal margin and the lateral border of the rectus muscle. It is frequently soft and diffuse, moving downwards on inspiration. If tender, the patient's inspiration is arrested with a gasp (Murphy's sign). This sign can be positive in the absence of gall bladder disease.

Courvoisier's Law. In the presence of jaundice a palpable gall bladder signifies carcinoma of the pancreas. If the jaundice is due to gallstones the gall bladder is fibrotic (chronic cholecystitis) and cannot distend. Consequently the gall bladder is impalpable. When carcinoma of the pancreas obstructs the common bile duct a normal gall bladder will distend. An exception to Courvoisier's law is a stone in the common bile duct associated with a stone in Hartman's pouch producing a mucocoele of the gall bladder.

Palpation of the spleen (surface markings, Figure 4)

The examiner leans across the patient and places his left hand behind the lower ribs. Palpation commences with the right hand in the left iliac fossa, the hand being advanced towards the left subcostal margin in the same manner as described under examination of the liver.

   If enlarged two to three times its normal size, the sharp lower border of the spleen will usually be felt medially to the anterior axillary line, though on occasions it is felt well lateral to this. In the presence of massive enlargement of the spleen the lower edge may cross the midline below the umbilicus. The following physical signs help to differentiate splenic from renal enlargement. The splenic notch

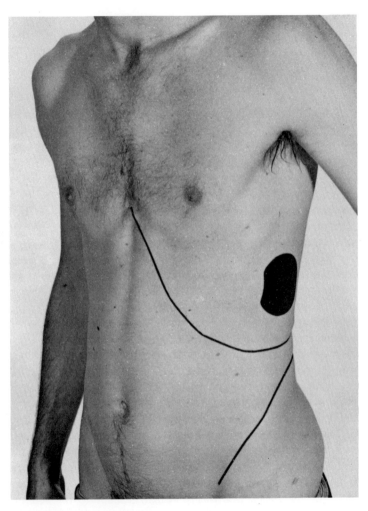

Fig. 4. The surface markings of the spleen. The spleen lies along the ninth, tenth and eleventh ribs in the posterior axillary line.

may be outlined by palpating along the medial border. With an enlarged spleen it is not possible to insert the hand between the spleen and the left costal border, while this is possible with renal enlargement. In addition, on percussing over the enlarged spleen dullness extends upwards to its normal surface markings which are along the ninth, tenth and eleventh ribs in the posterior axillary line. As a corollary to this, if the percussion note is resonant to the normal markings of the spleen there can be no significant splenic enlargement. When dullness to percussion suggests splenic enlargement the spleen may be more easily palpable if the patient rolls 30° towards the examiner and palpation is repeated commencing at the subcostal margin.

Causes of a palpable spleen

i. *Infective*
   a. Acute – viral hepatitis, glandular fever, septicaemia, bacteraemia
   b. Sub-acute – subacute bacterial endocarditis, brucellosis, typhoid fever
   c. Chronic – malaria.
ii. *Portal hypertension*
iii. *Haematological disorders.* Leukaemia, lymphomas, myelo-fibrosis, polycythaemia and haemolytic anaemias
iv. *Systemic disorders.* Disseminated lupus erythematosis, other collagen disorders, sarcoidosis
v. *Infiltrations.* Amyloid, lipid storage diseases e.g. Gaucher's disease.

Causes of massive enlargement of the spleen

i. Myelofibrosis
ii. Chronic leukaemia, especially chronic myeloid
iii. Giant follicular lymphoma
iv. Chronic malaria in indigenous peoples.

Palpation of the kidney

The left hand is placed posteriorly below the twelfth rib. Deep palpation begins at the level of the iliac crest with the fingers parallel to the rectus muscle. The palpating hand is advanced as described under examination of the liver. In a thin person the rounded lower pole of the right kidney may be palpable. An enlarged kidney may be ballotable, meaning that the kidney can be pushed from one examining hand to the other. However, a massively enlarged spleen is also ballotable.

Causes of bilaterally palpable kidneys
a. Polycystic disease
b. Bilateral hydro-nephrosis.

Causes of a unilateral palpable kidney
a. Polycystic disease with asymmetrical enlargement
b. Grawitz tumour
c. Hydro-or pyonephrosis
d. Displacement downwards of the kidney by an adrenal tumour
e. Solitary kidney
f. Normal right kidney.

While the kidneys may be enlarged in other conditions, such as nephrotic syndrome, leukaemia, amyloid disease, etc., they are rarely palpable.

Percussion of the abdomen

Percussion is used in conjunction with palpation in the identification of enlarged viscera. In the case of an enlarged impalpable liver it may be outlined by percussion. Similarly a distended bladder may be best identified by percussion downwards in the midline.

Auscultation of the abdomen

The following should be noted.

Bowel sounds

Normal bowel sounds are gurgling noises heard roughly every two to three seconds. If not heard at first they may be accentuated by flicking the abdomen in the flank. In ileus, bowel sounds are absent and in conditions associated with intestinal hurry or mechanical obstruction their frequency and loudness increases. With distension of the bowel, such as can occur in ulcerative colitis, the bowel sounds characteristically become tinkling.

Bruits

i. Renal artery stenosis. A bruit may be heard just above and to the left or right of the umbilicus, or occasionally posteriorly.
ii. Aneurysm of the aorta. A bruit may be heard in the epigastrium.
iii. Arterio-venous malformations and stenosis of other arteries may be associated with a bruit.
iv. Portal hypertension, in association with a large collateral venous circulation, may produce a venous hum in the epigastrium.

Friction rub

If heard over an enlarged spleen indicates infarction, while if heard over a large liver indicates malignancy or hepatic abscess.

AREA IDENTIFICATION
OF OTHER ABDOMINAL SWELLINGS

Swellings in the Right Iliac Fossa

i. *Appendiceal abscess.* A diffuse, tender, immobile swelling often associated with tenderness per rectum.
ii. *Carcinoma of the caecum.* A firm, localised, immobile and non-tender mass may be palpable.
iii. *Other causes.* Crohn's disease, tuberculosis and actinomycosis and these may be associated with external fistulae.

Swellings in the Left Iliac Fossa

i. *Descending colon.* If distended with faeces a sausage-shaped mass occurs which may be indented.
ii. *Carcinoma of the sigmoid or descending colon.* Usually a firm, localised, non-tender mass which does not move on respiration and is frequently immobile.
iii. *Diverticular disease of the sigmoid and descending colon.* May produce a similar mass, although if associated with inflammation it will be tender.

It should be emphasised that carcinoma of the sigmoid colon and diverticular disease rarely produce a palpable mass.

Swellings in the upper abdomen

i. *Aneurysm of the abdominal aorta.* A mass in the epigastrium which is immobile and frequently tender. Often only the left border is defined and when so is smooth and regular. Confirmatory evidence is expansile pulsation and a bruit.

ii. *Carcinoma of the stomach.* Rarely palpable, but if so a hard mass with an irregular edge which moves on respiration is felt in the epigastrium.

iii. *Pyloric stenosis.* The distended stomach is seen rather than felt in the upper abdomen. A gastric splash may be elicited by a sudden quick dipping movement of the hand over the distended area with the examiner's ear in close proximity to the abdomen. A gastric splash is significant only if the patient has not eaten within four hours. The cause of the stenosis is either chronic duodenal ulceration or carcinoma of the stomach. It is not to be confused with the infantile variety of pyloric stenosis.

iv. *Pancreatic tumour.* This rarely produces a palpable mass, but if so the mass is hard and immobile. A pseudo cyst of the pancreas may produce a diffuse or localised, tender, immobile swelling in the epigastrium.

v. *Retro-peritoneal masses.* Lymph node enlargement secondary to lymphoma is the commonest cause of a retroperitoneal mass and if palpable a firm, irregular and fixed mass is palpable in the region above the umbilicus. Enlarged lymph nodes secondary to testicular tumours may also be palpable in this region.

Pelvic Swellings

An immobile midline distension in the lower abdomen with a palpable upper border may be produced by a distended bladder, large ovarian cyst or a large uterus. The swelling of a distended bladder is relieved by catheterisation.

Examination of the genitalia and hernial orifices

The penis and scrotum should be inspected before the testes are palpated. The body of the testis on one side is compared with the other for size, shape, consistency and tenderness. Testicular swellings may be differentiated on the basis of translucency (a pocket torch is shone through the swelling from behind). Hydrocoeles and cysts of the epididymis, in particular, are translucent. The epididymis and spermatic cord are then palpated up to the superficial inguinal ring.

Inguinal and femoral herniae are best detected when the patient stands in front of the examiner. A visible impulse may be noted on coughing, and is frequently better seen than felt. The superficial inguinal ring is examined with the little finger being introduced by invaginating the scrotum with the finger nail lying against the spermatic cord. (Right hand for the right side and left hand for the left). The normal ring will just admit the tip of the little finger. When the finger is inserted, the patient is asked to cough to determine if there is a palpable expansile impulse, signifying a hernia. The bulge of a femoral hernia appears below the inguinal ligament and is more lateral than that of an inguinal hernia. Indirect inguinal herniae are more common than the direct form and appear at the superficial inguinal ring. Direct inguinal herniae appear medially through the inguinal triangle.

Digital examination of the rectum

The patient lies on his left side with the buttocks on the edge of the bed and the knees drawn up. The anus and peri-anal areas are inspected. This requires separation of the buttocks and good illumination. Inspection of the anus may reveal:
1. Ano-rectal fistulae
2. Ischio-rectal abscess
3. Skin tags
4. Thrombosed external haemorrhoids
5. Anal fissures
6. Excoriation from diarrhoea
7. Carcinoma of the anus
8. Rectal mucosal prolapse.

Then the gloved finger is lubricated and laid over the anus. With gentle backwards pressure the tip of the finger is inserted into the anal cavity and thence into the rectum. This procedure, although uncomfortable, is not painful and if pain occurs the following conditions are suggested – anal fissure, ischio-rectal abscess, proctitis, excoriation from diarrhoea or a recently thrombosed external haemorrhoid.

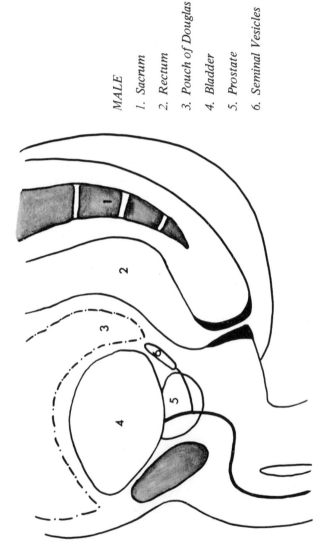

MALE
1. Sacrum
2. Rectum
3. Pouch of Douglas
4. Bladder
5. Prostate
6. Seminal Vesicles

Fig. 5a Anatomical landmarks identifiable on rectal examination.

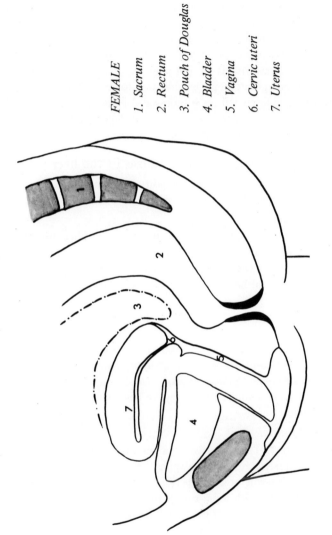

FEMALE
1. Sacrum
2. Rectum
3. Pouch of Douglas
4. Bladder
5. Vagina
6. Cervic uteri
7. Uterus

Fig. 5b Anatomical landmarks identifiable on rectal examination.

The rectal wall is examined by rotating the finger in a clockwise direction and feeling for intrinsic and extrinsic abnormalities, as indicated' in figure 5. Faeces in the rectum or sigmoid may be mistaken for a neoplasm as may a normal cervix uteri. It should be realised that haemorrhoids are not palpable unless thrombosed and therefore require proctoscopic examination to be diagnosed.

The finger is inspected on withdrawal for the presence of blood and the characteristics of the faeces are noted. A proctosigmoidoscopy should follow with biopsy where indicated.

Physical signs associated with cirrhosis of the liver

Cirrhosis of the liver may be present without any abnormal physical signs. However the following signs may occur.

Abdominal signs

i. *Hepatic size.* The liver may be enlarged and either smooth or irregular. Alternatively it may be small and then only be defined by percussion. In the presence of a hepatoma there may be a large nodule which can be painful and/or associated with a friction rub and/or bruit.

ii. *Splenic size.* An enlarged spleen indicates co-existing portal hypertension.

iii. *Dilated veins.* These may indicate portal hypertension.

iv. *Ascites.* Indicates a low serum albumin associated with portal hypertension or more rarely hepatic vein obstruction. If the serum albumin is low enough there may be co-existing oedema of the abdominal wall.

Extra abdominal signs

i. *Spider naevi.* These consist of a central dilated arteriole with radiating vessels resembling a spider, characteristically occurring in the distribution of the superior vena cava. Pressure over the central arteriole with a pin causes the whole angioma to blanch. In addition to cirrhosis of the liver naevi occur in normal subjects, pregnancy, thyrotoxicosis, rheumatoid arthritis and other collagen disorders.

ii. *Jaundice.* The bilirubin is usually less than 4 mg per 100 ml of blood and consequently is often only clinically detected in the sclerae. Higher levels of the serum bilirubin indicate severe hepatic decompensation.

iii. *Palmar erythema.* A reddish mottling of the thenar and hypothenar eminences of the hand. This also may occur in the same conditions as spider naevi.

iv. *Dupuytren's contractures.* Contractures of the palmar fascia occurring initially on the ulnar side of the hand, ultimately producing flexion deformities of the fingers. They are often more readily palpable than visible and are particularly associated with alcoholic cirrhosis.

v. *Bruising.* Commonly occurring on the extremities, due to trauma and associated with impaired clotting.

vi. *Bilateral parotid enlargement.* Painless and associated with alcoholic liver disease.

vii. *Generalised skin pigmentation.*

viii. *Endocrine.* Loss of body hair affecting particularly the face and axillae, testicular atrophy and gynaecomastia.

Other signs are described such as white nails, a high cardiac output state and cyanosis, but these are rarely of diagnostic clinical significance.

Additional characteristic physical signs occur with specific forms of cirrhosis.

i. *Biliary cirrhosis.* The jaundice may have a greenish tinge. Xanthomata occur, especially about the eyes. Scratch marks may be found on the skin.

ii. *Haemochromatosis.* Gross hepatomegaly, pigmentation, endocrine changes and glycosuria are common.

iii. *Cardiac cirrhosis.* Associated with signs of long standing cardiac failure usually secondary to mitral valve disease and tricuspid incompetence.

iv. *Wilson's disease.* Extrapyramidal neurological signs and Kayser-Fleischer rings may be present. A Kayser-Fleischer ring appears as a golden yellow ring situated near the circumference of the iris.

5

THE HAEMOPOIETIC SYSTEM

Abnormalities of the haemopoietic system may produce anaemia, polycythaemia, lymphadenopathy, hepatosplenomegaly or purpura, alone or in combination.

ANAEMIA

A. Pallor

This is the outstanding physical sign and is best confirmed by inspection of the conjunctivae and palmar creases. These should be inspected even in the absence of obvious facial pallor. To demonstrate pallor of the palmar creases the hand is hyper-extended, thus stretching these creases. If there is absence of the normal pinkish colour in the creases it is likely that the haemo-globin is under 8 gm per 100 ml of blood. For pallor of the hand to signify anaemia the hand should be warm and there should be associated pallor of the conjunctivae. The skin of the palms may appear pale without anaemia in the presence of callouses, shock and hypopituitarism. Red and inflamed conjunctivae may conceal the presence of anaemia.

B. Cardiovascular manifestations

Consist of a high output state with tachycardia and perhaps cardiac failure.

Causes of Anaemia

i. *Deficiency of factors necessary for blood production*
    a. Iron deficiency, including haemorrhage
    b. Vitamin B.12 deficiency
    c. Folate deficiency.

ii. *Depression of the bone marrow*
    a. Aplastic anaemia
    b. Bone marrow infiltration – leukaemia, malignant lymphoma, multiple myeloma, myelosclerosis and carcinoma
    c. Renal failure
    d. Infection
    e. Collagen disorders.

iii. *Increased red cell destruction (haemolytic anaemia)*
    a. Corpuscular defects – hereditary spherocytosis, thalassaemia and other haemoglobinopathies.
    b. Extracorpuscular defects (acquired haemolytic anaemias) associated with chronic lymphatic leukaemia, malignant lymphomas, collagen disorders and hypersplenism.

POLYCYTHAEMIA

If the face and mucous membranes appear plethoric, polycythaemia is suggested and should be confirmed by a haemoglobin estimation. A relative polycythaemia may occur in the presence of dehydration. The haemoglobin will then fall with subsequent rehydration.

Polycythaemia may be primary and then is usually associated with splenomegaly, or it may be secondary to a variety of disorders each with its own physical signs.

1. Cyanotic congenital heart disease
2. Respiratory failure
3. Renal disorders – carcinoma and hydronephrosis.

LYMPHADENOPATHY

Neck

Examination is first carried out from behind with the patient's neck flexed in order to relax the sternomastoid muscles. Lymphadenopathy may occur in relationship to the jugular vessels, submandibular and submental regions and anterior and posterior triangles of the neck. To examine the glands along the posterior border of the sterno-mastoids, occipital area, mastoid and pre-auricular regions, examination is best carried out from the front.

Axilla

This is first inspected with the patient's arm fully abducted. The examiner then places his hand in the axilla along the lateral chest wall and the patient fully adducts his arm and rests his forearm across the abdomen so that his pectoral muscles are relaxed. The examiner palpates the apical, posterior, anterior, medial and lateral areas of the axilla. In some cases the posterior group of axillary glands may be best palpated from behind.

Epitrochlear gland

The arm is relaxed and semi-flexed, the epitrochlear gland being identified just above the medial epicondyle in close relationship to the intermuscular septum between biceps and triceps muscles. The gland is best palpated using the thumb and forefinger.

The Groin

The glands lie along the inguinal ligament and in close relation to the femoral vessels.

In the presence of lymphadenopathy the following should be noted.
1. Situation.
2. Size and shape. Glands that are palpable but small do not necessarily indicate underlying disease.

3. Consistency. Glands infiltrated with secondary carcinoma are typically hard while lymphomatous glands are rubbery. Inflamed glands are soft and tender.
4. Discreteness. While any cause of lymphadenopathy may be associated with discrete lymph nodes, matting together of lymph nodes suggests lymphoma, malignant disease or tuberculosis.
5. Adherence to the skin or deep tissues suggests malignancy or tuberculosis.
6. Tenderness suggests inflammation.
7. Evidence of sinus formation or scarring occurs in tuberculosis and actinomycosis.

Causes of generalised lymphadenopathy

i. Infection — glandular fever
                rubella and other exanthemata
                toxoplasmosis
                tuberculosis
ii. Leukaemia
iii. Malignant lymphomas
iv. Carcinomatosis
v.   Collagen disorders
vi. Sarcoidosis.

Localised lymphadenopathy occurs as a reaction to local infections, but can be the precursor of generalised lymphadenopathy.

PURPURA

Purpuric spots are spontaneous petechiae or ecchymoses representing bleeding into or under the skin. They do not blanch on pressure and on fading leave a bluish discolouration as with a bruise. If present, the Hess test, an indicator of capillary fragility, should be carried out. The sphygmomanometer cuff is applied to the upper arm and inflated to a pressure midway between systolic and diastolic pressures for five minutes. It is then deflated and an area on the arm below the tourniquet which has previously been demarcated is inspected for the presence of fresh purpura. Purpura may be thrombocytopenic or non-thrombocytopenic and these are differentiated by performing a platelet count.

Causes of purpura

i. Thrombocytopenic
   idiopathic
   leukaemia
   aplastic anaemia
   bone marrow infiltration
   drugs
   collagen disorders
   hypersplenism
   systemic infections.

ii. Non-thrombocytopenic
   senile; this is usually not spontaneous and occurs on the backs of the hands
   uraemia
   diabetes
   polyarteritis nodosa
   systemic infections
   scurvy.

SPLENOMEGALY AND HEPATOMEGALY
(See pages 81 and 78)

Clinical Features of Leukaemia

1. Anaemia
2. Purpura (thrombocytopenic)
3. Infections (neutropenia). Ulceration in the mouth and pharynx, recurrent pneumonia and septicaemia
4. Sternal tenderness
5. Hepatosplenomegaly
6. Lymphadenopathy
7. Retinal haemorrhages and exudates
8. Skin infiltrations.

In acute leukaemia the only physical signs may be those due to lack of one or more of the three formed elements in the blood plus or minus sternal tenderness. In chronic leukaemia generalised enlargement of the lymph nodes, usually with hepatosplenomegaly, occurs. In chronic myeloid leukaemia the relative enlargement of the spleen is greater than that of the lymph nodes, while in chronic lymphocytic leukaemia the emphasis is on lymph node enlargement.

6

THE RESPIRATORY SYSTEM

Initially the following should be looked for: cyanosis (page 2); clubbing of the fingers (page 4) and whether the accessory muscles of respiration such as the sternomastoids and alae nasae are being used. The chest is then inspected preferably with the patient sitting upright or standing.

Inspection

1. *Shape of the chest*

   i. Normal. Flattened in the anterior posterior plane.

   ii. Barrel shaped. An increase in the anterior-posterior diameter together with a dorsal kyphosis. Expansion is limited and respiration is primarily diaphragmatic, the chest lifting upwards in inspiration. The presence of a barrel shaped chest is not a necessary prerequisite for making a diagnosis of emphysema.

   iii. Pigeon chest. A marked outward bowing of the upper sternum and costal cartilages.

   iv. Funnel chest. A depression of the lower end of the sternum.

   v. Deformities associated with kyphoscoliosis of the spine.

While the shape of the chest may be of no clinical significance, it can distort the underlying anatomy causing displacement of the apex beat, thus making assessment of cardiac size difficult.

2. *Rate and depth of respiration*

These are affected by:

i. Emotion which may produce tachypnoea or deep sighing respirations, either of which may ultimately result in tetany.

ii. Disturbance of pulmonary function produced by underlying lung or airways disease.

iii. Neurological disorders such as Guillain-Barré polyneuritis.

These disorders usually produce tachypnoea without an increase in depth of respiration. In airways obstruction prolonged inspiration and expiration may be evident, associated with audible wheezing.

iv. Changes in blood pH. Altered respiration occurs particularly in metabolic acidosis, there being an increase in depth and rate, provided there is normal pulmonary function.

3. *Chest expansion*

This is assessed with particular emphasis placed on any asymmetry. Asymmetry is best seen from the foot of the bed or from behind and above the patient looking down at the clavicles. An objective measurement can be obtained with a tape measure encircling the chest in the nipple line. Diminished movement on one side indicates underlying disease on that side.

4. *Position of the apex beat* (page 56)

Palpation

1. *The position of the mediastinum*

This is determined by locating the trachea and the apex beat.

Trachea. The index finger is advanced upwards and backwards over the mid point of the suprasternal notch and normally strikes the middle of the trachea. If displacement is present the finger will hit one or other side. Another method of assessing tracheal displacement is to run the index finger and middle fingers of the right hand down the medial sides of the sternomastoids. Normally the spaces on both sides of the trachea are equal.

Causes of tracheal displacement
a. Upper lobe fibrosis and/or atelectasis. Produces deviation towards the side of the lesion and this may be the only detectable sign.
b. Massive pleural effusion. Displacement away from the side of the lesion.
c. Pneumothorax. Displacement away from the side of the lesion.
d. Tumours of the upper mediastinum e.g. retrosternal goitre.
Apex beat. Respiratory causes of a displaced apex beat, in the presence of a normal heart, are those outlined above with the addition of collapse of a lower lobe causing displacement of the apex beat towards the side of the lesion.

2. **Chest movements**
The hands are positioned as shown in Figure 6a-d being firmly moulded to the chest wall, the thumbs being clear of the skin and in a relaxed position. The patient is asked to take a deep breath and expansion is gauged by the distance the thumbs move apart, any asymmetry of chest movement being noted. It should be emphasised that diminished movement implies an underlying lesion on that side.

3. **Vocal fremitus**
The hand is applied to the chest wall at the positions indicated in Figure 7, corresponding areas of each side of the chest being compared alternately. A characteristic vibration is felt when the patient says 99. Vocal fremitus is modified by the thickness of the chest wall and examination over the scapulae is misleading. Alterations in vocal fremitus are indicated in Table 1.

Percussion

The middle finger of the left hand is placed firmly along the intercostal space to be percussed and not across the ribs. The second phalanx is struck firmly by the right middle finger using a vertical action from the wrist. An intercostal space on one side is compared with that on the other. As with vocal fremitus, the percussion note is modified by the thickness of the chest wall. Alteration of the normal percussion

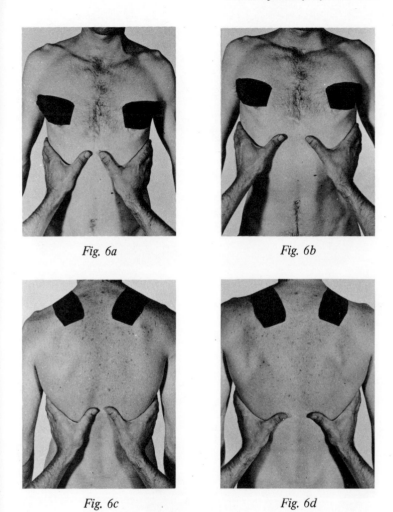

Fig. 6a

Fig. 6b

Fig. 6c

Fig. 6d

Fig. 6a, 6b, 6c & 6d. **Chest Movements**. *The hands are positioned anteriorly and posteriorly as shown. Figures a, c show the chest in expiration and figures 6, d in inspiration.*

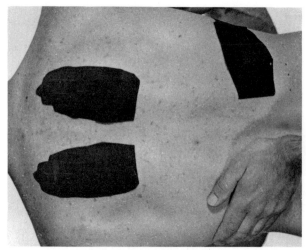

Fig. 7b

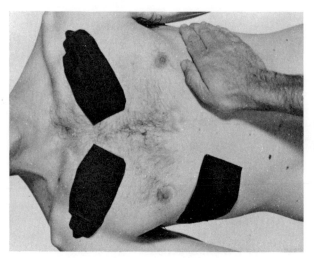

Fig. 7a

Fig. 7a & 7b. The hands are positioned as shown, care being taken to avoid assessing fremitus over the scapulae.

note is described as being hyper-resonant, hyporesonant or stony dull. Percussion is carried out in the areas shown in Figure 8 and if an abnormality is detected this area is carefully delineated. Percussion in the axilla is best carried out with the patient's hands placed on his head. Percussion over the scapulae is unreliable.

Liver dullness. The upper border of liver dullness occurs in the mid-clavicular line in the right fourth intercostal space or underlying the fifth rib, and in the axilla occurs in the sixth or seventh intercostal space.

Cardiac dullness. This is encountered in the third left intercostal space percussing downwards in the mid-clavicular line. The lateral border of the heart is located by percussing inwards along the fifth left interspace. Diminution of the normal area of liver and cardiac dullness may occur in emphysema.

Auscultation

The bell of the stethoscope is used, as friction against the diaphragm may produce false adventitious sounds. Again, right and left areas are compared alternately and auscultation is carried out in the areas indicated in Figure 8. If an abnormality is found then this area is delineated. During auscultation the patient breathes through the open mouth, taking only slightly deeper inspirations than normal to increase the loudness of the breath sounds. Distortion of the breath sounds occurs if inspiration is exaggerated.

Types of breath sounds

Vesicular. A soft blowing sound is heard throughout inspiration and through a third of expiration, without an intervening pause. The sound is louder in inspiration than expiration. Vesicular breathing is normally heard, except posteriorly between the scapulae and anteriorly under the clavicles, especially on the right, where the breathing is bronchovesicular.

Bronchial. A harsh blowing sound is heard throughout inspiration and expiration with an intervening pause. The sound in expiration is louder than that in inspiration. Bronchial breathing is heard over the trachea. Two variants of bronchial breathing are amphoric and

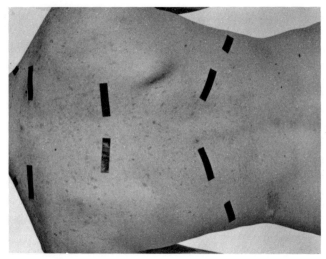

Fig. 8b

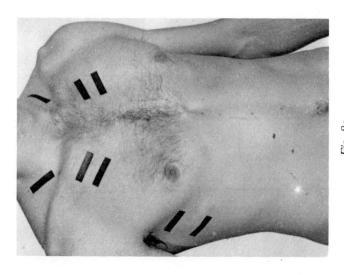

Fig. 8a

Fig. 8a & 8b. Percussion and auscultation are initially carried out in the areas indicated.

cavernous. These sounds may be heard over a cavity or pneumothorax. They may be simulated by blowing over a narrow or wide necked bottle respectively.

Bronchovesicular. This is intermediate between the above, the sound being heard throughout a greater part of expiration than in vesicular breathing and a pause being present.

Adventitious sounds

It should be realised that there is some confusion in the terminology of adventitious sounds. In addition too much emphasis should not be placed on minor variations in qualities of sound.

Crepitations. Discontinuous bursts of sounds heard mainly at the end of inspiration, resembling the crackling heard when the hair near the ear is rubbed between the fingers. Crepitations are not abolished by coughing. They reflect pathology in the alveoli or respiratory bronchioles, and characteristically occur in lobar pneumonia and diffuse interstitial fibrosis. In older people confined to bed a few basal crepitations may be heard, which usually but not invariably, disappear after a few breaths.

Râles. Harsher discontinuous sounds occurring more commonly in inspiration than expiration, reflecting bronchial pathology and characteristically occurring in bronchitis and pulmonary oedema.

Rhonchi. Continuous sounds heard either in expiration or inspiration being more common and louder in expiration. They reflect narrowing of larger order bronchi and may be high or low pitched, the former being typically heard in asthma. Low pitched rhonchi produced by mucus in major bronchi often disappear on coughing. Rhonchi may be diffuse as in asthma or localised and persistent and suggest a localised obstruction such as carcinoma of the bronchus.

Friction rub. A creaking noise of variable pitch produced by the rubbing together of pleural surfaces, being more commonly heard at the end of inspiration and in early expiration. Pleurisy of any cause, for example pneumonia or pulmonary infarction, may be associated with a rub.

Vocal resonance

The stethoscope is applied to the chest wall in the same areas as described under auscultation. The patient says 99 and the resonant sound is transmitted through the lung and chest wall. This sound may be increased or decreased as outlined in Table 1. If increased, the sign of whispering pectoriloquy may be elicited indicating underlying consolidation or cavitation. This is detected when the patient whispers 99, the words being then clearly audible through the stethoscope.

Many other auscultatory sounds have been described, but with the decline of cavitating tuberculosis these have little clinical relevance.

Inspection of the sputum

Sputum arises from the trachea, bronchi and lungs and should always be examined. The following abnormalities occur.

1. Mucoid sputum is whitish in colour, and is seen most frequently in chronic bronchitis and in asthma.

2. Muco-purulent sputum is creamy/green in colour and mixed with a varying amount of mucus. It signifies infection. Large amounts are produced daily in bronchiectasis and its odour may be offensive.

3. Purulent sputum is cream in colour and is seen following rupture of a lung abscess into a bronchus.

4. Blood-stained sputum (haemoptysis) occurs in:
   i. Carcinoma of the bronchus
   ii. Pulmonary embolus
   iii. Mitral stenosis
   iv. Left ventricular failure
   v. Tuberculosis
   vi. Infections including bronchiectasis.

   In acute pulmonary oedema, due usually to left ventricular failure or mitral valve disease, the sputum is watery, frothy, and may be blood-stained.

   Other types of sputum are described, but are rarely seen.

CORRELATION OF THE PHYSICAL SIGNS
WITH UNDERLYING PATHOLOGY

The first stage in diagnosis of respiratory disease is a combined pathological and anatomical one, e.g., consolidation of the left lower lobe. The second stage in diagnosis is aetiological and usually requires special investigations, e.g., pneumococcal lobar pneumonia involving the left lower lobe.

To make the first stage diagnosis it should be asked whether the physical signs elicited correspond to any primary type of pathology. However, it is important to realise that all physical signs may not be present and in fact the diagnosis may be made on one physical sign alone, for example, deviation of the trachea indicating fibrosis of an upper lobe.

The physical signs of the first stage diagnosis are outlined in Table 1.

In addition to the physical signs outlined in Table 1 there are certain additional features described below.

Consolidation

In the early stage of consolidation breath sounds may be diminished before they become bronchial. Bronchial breath sounds may be the only sign of underlying consolidation. A pleural friction rub may or may not be heard and crepitations often only become apparent during the healing stage. In broncho-pneumonia the signs are usually bilateral and may be associated with rhonchi indicating underlying bronchitis. The aetiological agent in lobar pneumonia is usually the pneumococcus while in broncho-pneumonia the common organisms are haemophilus influenzae and pneumococci.

Pleural Effusion

Clinically detectable mediastinal shift towards the opposite side occurs only with large effusions. The apex beat is usually impalpable in a left sided effusion and the right border of the heart may be detected by percussion to the right of the sternum in the fourth intercostal space. In a right sided effusion the apex beat may be displaced to the left. Only massive effusions produce deviation of the trachea. While the physical signs of consolidation may occur above an effusion they do not necessarily indicate underlying pneumonia and the mechanism for their production is controversial. Dullness to percussion occurs both with a pleural effusion and with consolidation; however, in the case of a pleural effusion the dullness extends higher in the axilla than posteriorly (Ellis's S-shaped line). This occurs because fluid in the pleural cavity does not follow surface markings of the major lobes of the lung. Ellis's line disappears when there is air above the fluid, such as commonly occurs following a paracentesis.

Causes

i. Cardiac failure
ii. Pneumonia
iii. Malignancy, e.g., carcinoma of the bronchus, lymphoma
iv. Pulmonary embolus
v. Tuberculosis
vi. Hypoalbuminaemia, e.g., cirrhosis of the liver, nephrotic syndrome.

The definitive diagnosis depends on the history, other physical signs such as Horner's syndrome, clubbing of the fingers, hypertrophic pulmonary osteoarthropathy etc. and often on further investigation by sputum examination, radiology and bronchoscopy. Paracentesis followed by a further chest X-ray may reveal pathology in the lung previously obscured by the fluid.

Collapse

Collapse and consolidation often coexist. Whilst collapse may be due to compression of the lung by a large pleural effusion or pneumothorax, the signs are those of the latter. The term "collapse" usually implies bronchial obstruction, secondary to carcinoma of the bronchus or an inhaled foreign body.

Fibrosis

This is almost invariably confined to the upper lobe and when long standing is associated with flattening of the chest. The only common cause is tuberculosis.

Diffuse interstitial fibrosis is a different entity, the classical physical sign being bilateral, symmetrical coarse basal crepitations.

Pneumothorax

Diminished movement is the important sign as hyperresonance is difficult to distinguish from normal resonance. Indeed, the percussion note on the normal side may be considered hyporesonant. Deviation of the trachea only occurs with a tension pneumothorax. Occasionally a systolic click is heard with a left sided pneumothorax.

Pneumothoraces are commonly spontaneous and not associated with underlying gross pathology. However, a pneumothorax can complicate underlying pulmonary conditions such as emphysema, asthma, tuberculosis, carcinoma, etc. A pneumothorax is common in chest injuries when haemothorax usually co-exists.

Emphysema

The signs are due to loss of pulmonary elastic recoil with disruption of alveoli and bronchial narrowing especially in expiration. Total lung volume is increased and cardiac and liver dullness may be diminished. Breath sounds are decreased. Crepitations and râles are not a feature but expiratory rhonchi may be present.

Airways obstruction

This is commonly due to chronic, acute, or acute on chronic bronchial disease due to irritants (e.g. cigarette smoke) or infection. It is the cardinal feature of bronchial asthma. Obstruction is greater in expiration than in inspiration and the chest becomes overinflated as in emphysema, with which airway obstruction is usually confused. Râles and rhonchi are prominent. In acute exacerbations pulmonary gas exchange is severely compromised resulting in hypoxia (cyanosis) and hypercapnia due to disturbance of normal ventilation − perfusion relationships.

Mediastinal compression

The integrity of mediastinal structures may be compromised by a variety of pathological processes.

1. Enlargement of lymph nodes secondary to carcinoma of the bronchus or malignant lymphomas
2. Enlargement of a retrosternal thyroid gland or thymus
3. Aneurysm of the aorta.

   The physical signs associated with mediastinal compression are:

1. *Superior vena cava obstruction*

   This is manifest by:

   i. Non pulsating engorgement of the jugular veins
   ii. Oedema of the head, neck and arms which often makes the engorged jugular veins difficult to see
   iii. Cyanosis of the above areas
   iv. Dilated collateral veins over the chest
   v. Papilloedema.

   In partial obstruction not all these signs are present.

2. *Compression of the trachea*

   An audible, harsh inspiratory sound (stridor) often associated with respiratory distress.

3. *Compression of the oesophagus*

   Progressive dysphagia for solids.

4. *Involvement of the left recurrent laryngeal nerve*

   Hoarseness of the voice.

5. *Involvement of the sympathetic pathways*

   Horner's syndrome.

   i. Lack of facial sweating on the affected side
   ii. Meiosis
   iii. Ptosis
   iv. Enophthalmos

6. *Paralysis of the phrenic nerve*

   While paradoxical movements of the diaphragm may sometimes be demonstrated by retraction of the epigastrium on the affected side during inspiration the only reliable sign is lack of diaphragmatic movement shown by radiological screening.

TABLE 1　The physical signs associated with LEFT SIDED pulmonary pathology

	Mediastinal Position	Movement on the side of the lesion	Percussion Note	Breath Sounds	Vocal Fremitus	Vocal Resonance	Adventitious Sounds
Consolidation	Normal	Decreased	Hypo-resonant	Bronchial	Increased	Increased	Crepitations Friction rub
Effusion	Normal or deviated to right	Decreased	Stony dull	Diminished or absent	Diminished or absent	Absent	Variable
Collapse	Deviated to left	Decreased	Hypo-resonant	Bronchial or absent	Increased or decreased	Increased or decreased	Variable
Fibrosis	Deviated to left	Decreased	Hypo-resonant	Bronchial or absent	Increased or decreased	Increased or decreased	Variable
Pneumothorax	Deviated to right	Decreased	Hyper-resonant	Diminished absent or Amphoric	Decreased	Decreased	—
Emphysema	Normal	Decreased	Resonant	Diminished	Decreased	Decreased	Rhonchi
Airways Obstruction	Normal	Decreased	Resonant	Variable	Decreased	Decreased	Rhonchi Râles

7

THE ENDOCRINE SYSTEM

The clue to the presence of endocrine disorders is often given by the appearance of the patient; consequently these disorders may be missed unless specifically thought of at the initial interview. The following common endocrine disorders occur.

Thyrotoxicosis

The general appearance of the patient is often striking in that he is agitated, restless, speaks rapidly, is emotionally labile, pigmented, has prominent staring eyes and may clearly have lost weight. However, all these overt signs of thyrotoxicosis may be absent in the elderly patient in whom only the cardiovascular manifestations occur.

The thyroid gland

May be visibly enlarged (goitre) and is examined from behind with the patient's neck slightly flexed to relax the sterno-mastoid muscles. Both lobes of the thyroid and the isthmus are defined by palpation, care being taken to get below the lower limit of the thyroid gland to exclude a retrosternal extension. If this is not possible a retrosternal extension may be outlined by percussion. The features to be noted on palpation are whether the gland is smooth or nodular and whether the enlargement is symmetrical. If nodular, the gland is usually firm, but if diffusely enlarged it is soft and may be tender.

Any locally enlarged lymph nodes should be noted. An enlargement in the neck that moves up and down on swallowing confirms that it is thyroid in origin. Both lobes of the thyroid gland are then auscultated for the presence of a continuous murmur which may be accompanied by a thrill; if present these indicate hyper-activity of the gland. A systolic murmur may be audible, but is transmitted from the aortic area through the carotid arteries and does not imply hyperthyroidism. Thyrotoxicosis may be present without thyroid gland enlargement, particularly in the elderly.

A variety of *eye signs* may be associated.

Associated eye signs

Lid retraction. The upper lids are retracted so that a small area of sclera is seen above the iris.

Lid lag. The patient is asked to look at the examiner's finger which is held at least two feet from the patient's eyes and moved slowly down from above. In the presence of lid lag delay in the upper lids following the movement of the eyeballs downwards reveals the white sclera above the iris.

Exophthalmos. There is protrusion of the eyes which is usually bilateral but may be unilateral. It is first apparent by the sclera becoming visible below and later above the iris. Severe exophthalmos may be associated with conjunctivitis and chemosis (conjunctival oedema).

Ophthalmoplegia. The patient complains of diplopia and this is tested for as described on page 18.

In addition to the above eye signs the hands are warm and sweaty and the nails may show the presence of onycholysis. A *fine tremor* may be demonstrated in the outstretched hands. The tremor is accentuated by placing a sheet of paper on the dorsum of the hand with the fingers separated. A *proximal myopathy* is common and is manifest by weakness and wasting in the limb girdles and neck flexors. Thickening of the skin which is reddened, cool and hairless, may be found over the lateral lower leg — pre-tibial myxoedema. It occurs only in association with eye signs.

Associated cardiovascular signs

i. Sustained tachycardia and systolic hypertension
ii. Atrial fibrillation and/or cardiac failure, the latter rarely occurring in the absence of fibrillation.

Myxoedema

Early changes of myxoedema are subtle and easily overlooked and the following gross changes are only apparent late in the course of the disease. The facial appearance becomes characteristic with baggy eyelids and a puffy face which may also be sallow or have a reddish tinge due to carotenaemia. The hair is dry and brittle, and the outer third of the eyebrows may be sparse. The skin of the face and hands is strikingly dry and cool. There is slowness of speech and thought associated with a husky voice.

The thyroid gland may not be palpable, but is sometimes enlarged, firm and woody (Hashimoto's thyroiditis).

The reflexes, particularly the ankle jerks, may be myotonic, in that there is a brisk contraction of the muscle with slow relaxation. The patient may be drowsy and in fact present in coma with associated hypothermia. Cerebellar signs may also occur.

The cardiovascular signs are sinus bradycardia and cardiac enlargement with cardiac failure secondary to ischaemic heart disease. A pericardial effusion occasionally occurs.

Addison's disease

The patient appears asthenic and may be dehydrated following vomiting associated with abdominal pain. Hypotension is universal and there is a fall in systolic blood pressure on standing.

Pigmentation is common and characteristically occurs in the mucous membranes of the mouth and hard palate. It is also present in scars and in pressure areas such as the elbows, knees and belt line. When present it is more prominent in exposed areas.

Cushing's syndrome

The facial appearance is characteristic, being plethoric and puffy.

Signs of masculinization may be present – hirsutism and acne. There is associated obesity, particularly of the trunk, with pads of fat in the supra-clavicular regions and over the upper thoracic spine (buffalo hump). Due to the rapid increase in weight reddened striae appear over the abdomen and buttocks; similar striae are seen in pregnancy and with rapid weight gain in obese patients. Generalised weakness, a proximal myopathy, fragility of the skin manifest by bruising, peripheral oedema and systemic hypertension occur. Dorsal kyphosis or vertebral collapse may occur secondary to osteoporosis.

Acromegaly

The face appears leonine with prominence of the lower jaw and widening of the spaces between the teeth. The hands and feet are also enlarged as are other organs such as the thyroid, heart, liver and spleen and the skin may appear coarse. Bi-temporal hemianopia or ultimately blindness in one or both eyes may follow pressure on the optic chiasm by the pituitary adenoma. Glycosuria consequent upon hyperglycaemia occurs.

Hypopituitarism

The skin is thin, cool and pale with absence of body hair and a poor beard growth in the male. Signs of hypothyroidism, adrenal insufficiency and gonadal insufficiency may be associated.

Hypoparathyroidism

The prominent features are neuromuscular hyper-excitability and tetany. Tetany is a painful spasm of the hands and feet which can arise spontaneously or be provoked by ischaemia of the limb (Trousseau's sign). To elicit this the blood pressure cuff is inflated to midway between systolic and diastolic pressures for three minutes. Tapping with the finger over the branches of the facial nerve may produce flickering of the corner of the mouth (Chvostek's sign).

8

EXAMINATION OF JOINTS

The following is a general scheme for the examination of joints which should be inspected and palpated for:

1. The presence of swelling and/or deformity which may be due to:
   i. Fluid (effusion). Fluctuation may be detected by placing the two index fingers one to two centimetres apart over the swelling. On pressing one finger down the other finger will rise. In the presence of an effusion into the knee joint, a *patellar tap* may be elicited by firmly grasping and suddenly depressing the patella against the lower end of the femur. This produces a sensation of moving through fluid before tapping the bone.
   ii. Bone outgrowths. Characteristic of osteoarthritis, but can occur in any proliferative arthropathy. A common site of occurrence is at the sides of the terminal interphalangeal joints of the fingers (Heberden's nodes).
   iii. Bursae. Enlargement of bursae does not necessarily mean underlying arthropathy and commonly occurs following repeated trauma, for example over the olecranon and knee.
   iv. Thickening of the synovial membrane and periarticular tissue.
2. Distribution of the arthropathy. Is it monarticular or polyarticular; are small and/or large joints affected and is the arthropathy symmetrical or asymmetrical.
3. Local muscle wasting.

4. Associated features. *Gouty tophi,* which are firm, non-tender, palpable, whitish deposits occurring in the periarticular areas and the cartilage of the ear. They may ulcerate through the skin and extrude a chalky-looking material (urate crystals). *Nodules,* subcutaneous, firm, non-tender, circumscribed nodules occurring in periarticular regions and over tendons in rheumatoid arthritis and gout.
5. Range of movement. This is estimated by putting the joint through a range of passive movements. The degree of limitation is assessed by comparison with unaffected joints or by a knowledge of normal joint movement. Limitation of movement may be due to pain, muscle spasm, effusion, joint disruption and muscle contracture.

ARTHROPATHIES

Rheumatoid arthritis

A symmetrical arthritis involving small and large joints. In the hand it classically involves the proximal interphalangeal joints with sparing of the distal interphalangeal joints. There may be associated nodules and bursae. Subluxation of the joints and ulnar deviation of the fingers may occur as late phenomena. In psoriasis there may be an arthritis which resembles rheumatoid arthritis, the additional features being involvement of the distal interphalangeal joints and psoriatic changes in the nails. A rheumatoid type of arthritis associated with clubbing of the fingers occurs in carcinoma of the lung (hypertrophic pulmonary osteoarthropathy).

Gout

Acute gout is typically monarticular, the joint being swollen, red, oedematous and exquisitely tender, resembling cellulitis. It classically affects the first metatarso-phalangeal joint.

Chronic tophaceous gout is typically polyarticular and asymmetrical, involving any joint. It may be associated with tophi, nodules and bursae.

Osteoarthritis

Large, weight bearing joints such as the knees, hips, and ankles are typically involved. Obesity is a common associated problem and the joints may have previously been damaged by trauma.

There occurs a proliferative, destructive arthritis in which there is an excessive range of painless movement (at least in one direction) seen in syphilis and diabetes — a Charcot joint.

INDEX